TRANC

TRANQUILLIZERS

The Comprehensive Guide

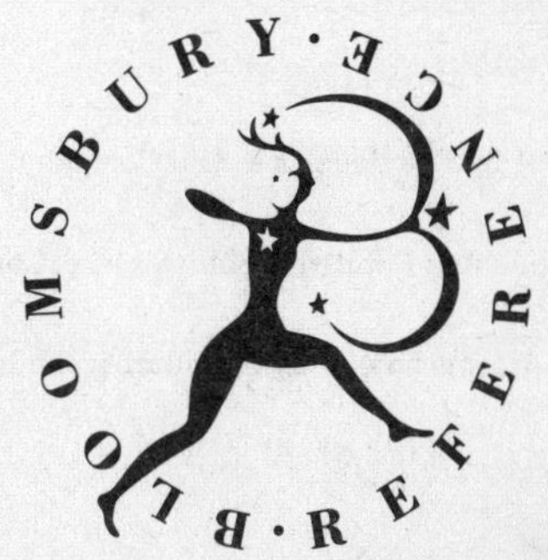

BLOOMSBURY

CONSULTANTS AND CONTRIBUTORS

Dr Ian K.M. Morton BSc, PhD, *King's College London*
(Series Consultant)
Dr John Halliday BSc, PhD, *King's College London*
(Consultant Editor)
Dr Judith M. Hall BSc, PhD, *King's College London*
(Technical Editor)

While the creators of this work have made every effort to be as accurate and up-to-date as possible, medical and pharmaceutical knowledge is constantly changing and the application of it to particular circumstances depends on many factors. Therefore readers are urged always to consult a qualified medical specialist for individual advice. The contributors, editors, consultants and publishers of this book can not be held liable for any errors and omissions, or actions that may be taken as a consequence of using it.

First published 1992

Bloomsbury Publishing Limited, 2 Soho Square, London W1V 5DE

The CIP record for this book is available from the British Library.

ISBN 0 7475 0994 8

Designed by Malcolm Smythe
Typeset by August Filmsetting, St Helens
Printed in Great Britain by
Cox & Wyman Ltd, Reading

CONTENTS

PREFACE

This dictionary is a comprehensive guide to the range of medicines, available in the United Kingdom today, that affect some aspect of the workings of the brain. It is not intended to be a guide to the prescription or administration of drugs; a qualified practitioner should always be consulted before any medicine is taken.

What is this book about?

There are many types of drug that affect some aspect of the workings of the brain. This book sets out to provide information on those drugs that are used in conventional medical practice. It is not the intention of this dictionary to deal with the many mind-altering drugs that are only used socially, such as alcohol or the nicotine in cigarettes, or the non-medical uses of drugs (such as the narcotic heroin) which are also in medical use. There is, however, some mention of drugs used to treat substance dependence.

The A to Z section of the book details, under name headings, both individual medical drugs ('medicines') in use in the UK, together with entries giving condensed information on relevant classes of these drugs. Among the more important of the classes explained are the MINOR TRANQUILLIZERS and the MAJOR TRANQUILLIZERS (used to treat anxiety and psychotic states, respectively), ANTIDEPRESSANT drugs of various types (used to treat depressive states), and ANALGESICS (which are used in the alleviation of pain). A number of other drugs classes are also covered, and these are as varied as ANTI-EPILEPTIC and ANTIPARKINSONIAN drugs, HYPNOTIC drugs (which promote sleep), and GENERAL ANAESTHETICS. We do not deal with drugs that are used to treat infections affecting the brain (e.g. meningitis), nor those used to treat tumours which may affect brain function.

The Introduction of the book will help readers who wish to understand in more detail how the drugs work. Topics include the workings of the brain, its disturbance in disease states, and its modification by drugs. There are detailed entries on the major drug classes and discussion of the use and safety of drugs, which expand on the information given in the A to Z entries.

For whom is this book intended

It is hoped that there is much in this book for many different people. Some sections of the Introduction, and some entries in the A to Z, are sufficiently technical to be of value to those concerned with health care or training for a medical or paramedical qualification. Overall though, it is hoped that there is sufficient cross-referencing of entries, and help from the explanations relating to drugs classes and their uses in the Introduction, to allow someone without a technical background to gain important information about which drugs are used for what purpose. There can be few people who have not themselves taken, or had friends or family use, medicines of the types described in this dictionary, whether by prescription or from over-the-counter sale. For those who wish to relate the proprietary names of drugs they are prescribed to the generic drug, or who are interested in the side-effects of the drugs and the circumstances in which they should and should not be used, the book may also be of value. For those who are experiencing at first hand the traumas of the treatment of someone for whom they care, it is hoped there may be sufficient information to allow a better understanding of the main actions and possible side-effects of the drugs involved. However, in no way is this book intended as a guide to self-medication (and thus there is no mention of dosage). However, it should make the choice of, for example, a proprietary analgesic preparation for headaches and minor pains somewhat simpler (and safer), by uncovering the rather confusing relationship between the proprietary name and the constituent active generic drug(s) that it contains.

How to use this book

The book is divided into sections. It begins with an Introduction that gives some background information on medical disorders that affect the brain and of the types of medicinal drugs that are used in their treatment.

The main A to Z section of the book contains entries that describe the medicinal drugs available. The drugs are listed under their generic and their proprietary names. There are also articles covering the major drug types (indicated by *). The A to Z is thoroughly cross-referenced. Cross-references are indicated by SMALL CAPITALS. Many of the articles detail the possible side-effects (indicated by ●) and list warnings (indicated ▲) to be borne in mind when administering a particular drug.

Drugs are usually named in one of two ways. The generic name (without an initial capital letter) is the official chemical name, and should describe the active constituent regardless of the source of the drug. The proprietary name (with an initial capital letter) is a brand name, a preparation of a drug, or mixture of drugs, that represents a particular formulation from a given manufacturer.

Doctors are encouraged to prescribe drugs using the generic name, because it is simpler and cheaper. Established drugs are often available as a standard preparation; for instance *paracetamol B.P.* must be formulated as laid down in the British Pharmacopoeia. This ensures that it dissolves within a certain time and contains a precise amount of the active chemical. More or less the same preparation is available under a number of different proprietary names, and they are generally more expensive. However, when a new drug is first introduced it is commonly protected by a patent granted to a single manufacturer or distributor, and the proprietary and generic preparation will be identical. Although the method of description will differ, the actual packaging will generally show both names, but with prominence given to the proprietary name. When the patent expires, if the drug is still believed to be of value, several manufacturers may market the same generic drug, either as a generic, or under their own proprietary names (often with small differences in formulation, such as sustained-release tablets).

These arrangements with two or more names for the same drug are, of course, complicated. A number of authoritative listings of drugs have evolved; each has its particular usage, particularly in respect of official or authoritative accounts of dosage, side-effects, indications and contra-indications according to disease state, interactions with other drugs, and other technical matters. This book is not a substitute for these professional guides, but represents a synopsis of some of their contents (more details may be found in the publications listed below).

Established preparations are described in the British Pharmacopoeia and Martindale's Extra Pharmacopoeia. The British National Formulary (BNF) is an impartial guide prepared jointly by the British Medical Association and the Royal Pharmaceutical Society of Great Britain. It is revised twice yearly, and is distributed free to hospital doctors. The Monthly Index of Medical Specialities (MIMS) is a listing of proprietary drugs and is distributed mainly to General Practitioners. The ABPI Handbook (Association of the British Pharmaceutical Industry) is a compendium of detailed data sheets on proprietary preparations. A critique of selected current drugs is given fortnightly in Drugs and Therapeutics Bulletin (Consumers Association), and there are selected articles on the side-effects of drugs in Adverse Drug Reactions Bulletin (Meditext).

Even with this number of publications it is difficult to keep the prescriber of drugs up to date, and there are advantages in using computer database equivalents in hospitals and in general practice. A further problem in promptly warning prescribers about newly reported adverse effects of drugs, which are monitored by 'yellow forms' sent in by doctors to the Committee on Safety of Medicines (or now, the Medicines Control Agency).

These points indicate the unceasing change that occurs in the drug industry and medical research, making pharmacology and therapeutics a science that requires expert and up-to-date information and evaluation.

Dr Ian K. M. Morton
Series consultant

INTRODUCTION

THE ORIGINS OF DRUGS THAT AFFECT THE MIND

It is not really surprising that the introduction to this book needs, at the outset, to make some distinction between the medical use of chemicals that affect the mind, and the social, religious or illegal use of these and similar drugs. It is clear that mankind has always sought out with special enthusiasm agents that modify consciousness or the state of mind in some pleasurable way. For instance, probably every race on earth has learned to brew alcoholic beverages, and remains of opium poppies have been found at the sites of the earliest societies. In various continents of the world, these and many other vegetable products containing drugs with powerful effects on the mind were discovered early: these include coca leaves (COCAINE), tobacco (NICOTINE), hashish (marijuana – CANNABIS), opium (MORPHINE), mushroom extracts (various hallucinogenic substances), and other natural psychoactive substances.

It is certain that pharmacology has learned much from this earlier experimentation and that a number of such chemicals (e.g. morphine) are still used in medicine. It is also true that this knowledge has exacted its price. Indeed, the motivation behind the primitive investigation of natural psychoactive plant extracts seems to have been largely to discover agents that could induce 'chemical vacations', away from or beyond reality. It is perhaps ironic therefore that some of the most challenging objectives in pharmacology today are to discover drugs that can help psychiatrists in their efforts to do the opposite, namely, return towards normality those minds that are too disturbed or distracted for the individual to play a normal part in society.

Any historian trying to establish a perspective on the 'drug abuse' problems of our current Western society will be aware how the utilization of these largely plant substances has developed in many cases from being an art (jealously guarded, for example, by witch-doctors, or members of esoteric societies) to something readily available by any who can pay the market price. In some cultures it may be difficult to separate the 'social' uses from the 'medical' uses. However, in the UK, legislation distinguishes between the beneficial medical, and the harmful social use of drugs such as morphine, amphetamines, and barbiturates.

Medicinal drugs that act on the brain have, by the late 20th century, become very big business. Prescriptions for such drugs make up one of the biggest drug bills in the NHS. It might be imagined from this massive prescribing that the science of these drugs is well advanced. However, in many cases the detailed mode of action of the drug is poorly understood, though the overall effects of the drug in health or disease may be reasonably clear. This undoubtedly reflects our very imperfect understanding of how the brain itself works. Indeed, predictions of 25 years ago by some in the medical community, that it was only a matter of years before the drugs to conquer mental illness would be developed, have proved wildly over-optimistic. Nevertheless, recent advances in our understanding of brain function at the cellular or molecular level do hold out genuine cause for hope of a new generation of more selective drugs with fewer and less intrusive side-effects.

THE MIND, THE BRAIN AND THE CENTRAL NERVOUS SYSTEM

Before going on to outline some ways in which the brain can 'go wrong', and how drugs act to exert a beneficial effect, it may be helpful to consider some aspects of the function of the brain, and the nerves that serve it.

From a simple point of view the brain can be thought of as the thinking and controlling centre of the body. The neuroscientist distinguishes between the *central nervous system* (this being made up of the brain and the spinal cord) and the *peripheral nervous system* (this being made up of the sensory and motor nerves running from the brain or spinal cord to tissues such as muscle, the heart, blood vessels and the skin). In this book we will be concerned primarily with drugs affecting the central nervous system. The *spinal cord* acts as a conduit for nerves to and from the brain and provides the location of many basic levels of reflex control. The *brain* is the site of higher-order functions such as the integration of complex voluntary movements (involved, for example, in speech or playing a musical instrument), the special senses (such as vision and hearing), feelings (like anxiety, pain, or pleasure), and indeed, of thought itself.

To all intents and purposes therefore, the brain can be described as the seat of the mind. Drugs affecting the *mind* (or *psyche*) are often termed *psychoactive* or *psychotropic* agents; and hallucinogens and ANTIDEPRESSANTS would serve as examples of such drugs. Other drugs (such as ANTI-EPILEPTICS and ANTIPARKINSONIAN drugs) are not used primarily for their effect on the mind, but rather for their effect on brain functions not directly involving the psyche (e.g. control of muscle tone). Such drugs could be said to be used to treat *neurological* conditions of the brain, that is, those in which there is good evidence of an underlying organic defect in the structure or basic operating system of the brain. This distinction between neurological and psychiatric disorders of the brain is far from absolute, but it is operationally useful.

The brain and its chemistry

In this century it has been recognised that the brain operates as a complex interconnecting network of nerve cells. Each of these individual nerve cells (or *neurones* as they are called) has the capacity to become active (*excited*), generating and conducting a very small electrical impulse along its length untl it terminates on a receptive area on another neurone. The arrival of such an impulse, an *action potential*, at a nerve terminal causes the release of a minute amount of a *neurotransmitter*, a chemical specific to that particular type of nerve cell. This neurotransmitter then diffuses across the small *synaptic gap* between neurones to act on *receptors* on the next nerve cell in the circuit, to excite or to inhibit it. This process is known as *synaptic transmission*. Signals passing from neurone to neurone in this way generate patterns of activity in a multitude of circuits which in some mysterious way endow the individual with the ability to generate what we call sensations, emotions, or thoughts. Following from this, the brain may initiate remote actions such as contraction of muscles giving rise to movements of the body, or at a more basic (involuntary or *autonomic*) level it may bring about an increase in heart-rate or an increase in sweating. All this is made possible by the process of *chemical neurotransmission* between neurones, whereby a chemical released from an active neurone binds to and activates receptors on a target neurone, either activating or inhibiting the target neurone. This signalling takes place at very distinct sites (*synapses*) and one single neurone may receive input from many other neurones through multiple synaptic contacts. The neurone may in turn, through branching of its terminals, synapse on many other neurones.

It is the particular concern of the neuropharmacologist to find chemicals, natural or synthetic, that can inhibit, mimic, or potentiate this natural process of synaptic neurotransmission. But, one might ask, how does this relate to the psychoactive properties of drugs? Through advances in neuroscience in the last half-century it has become clear that most drugs with profound actions on the brain interfere in some way with synaptic neurotransmission. To take an example – all the major ANTIPSYCHOTIC drugs (major tranquillizers) are now recognised to inhibit the effects of a particular set of nerve cells in the brain, which bring about their actions by the release of the chemical neurotransmitter DOPAMINE. On the other hand, all agents such as AMPHETAMINE or COCAINE, which potentiate or cause the release of dopamine from dopaminergic neurones in the brain, have stimulatory effects on the mind. Similar evidence has accumulated for other neurotransmitters, suggesting links between individual neurotransmitters and particular brain activities or states.

What can go wrong with brain function?

The various disorders of the brain may be placed in certain classes. One class, often termed neurological, refers to situations in which there is clear evidence of a physical abnormality or damage to the tissues of the brain. Such abnormalities may be congenital (e.g. *spina bifida*; or *Down's syndrome*), or the damage may be caused by a severe viral (e.g. *viral encephalitis*) or bacterial (e.g. *meningitis*; brain abscess) infection affecting the brain. Other frequent causes of neurological damage are *trauma* (e.g. a wound to the head in a car accident), *tumours* (malignant and non-malignant), and *strokes* (caused either by blockage of major blood vessels in the brain, or by haemorrhage from the vessels, leading in either case to a failure in the blood supply and death of the nervous tissue in the affected area of distribution). *Epilepsy* is classed as a neurological disorder even though the specific nature of the physical damage to the brain is often unknown. *Multiple sclerosis* is another relatively common neurological disorder caused by the destruction of non-neural cells which normally support and nourish nerve cells in the brain and spinal cord. Without this support these nerve cells fail to conduct impulses in the normal manner.

Another important class of disorder of the brain covers the degenerative conditions in which there is relatively specific neurodegeneration affecting characteristic nerve cells in the brain. For instance, *Parkinson's disease*, *Alzheimer's disease* and *Huntington's chorea* are all conditions in which specific patterns of neurodegeneration are seen, and as a result of which characteristic symptoms develop.

The final class of disorder to be considered in this introduction are the psychiatric states including such examples as *clinical depression, incapacitating anxiety, manic depression, personality disorders* and *acute* or *chronic psychotic states*, the latter being most commonly encountered in *schizophrenia*. These are all conditions that primarily affect the higher-order functions of the brain, and are usually associated with readily recognisable abnormalities of mood, emotion, sensation, or thoughts. The cause of such disorders is little understood. Some, usually of the *psychoanalytical school*, have emphasised the role of early and unresolved conflicts between the conscious and the unconscious mind. Others of the *behaviourist school* would point to the importance of previous experience in conditioning present behaviour. Others again, of the *organic school*, might look for a more physical explanation such as over-activity in a particular nerve circuit. The problem of establishing causation in such cases is very much a chicken-and-egg situation. Did the defective 'circuit' cause the defective behaviour or did the pattern of behaviour modify the 'circuit'? As yet, neuroscience is unable to answer these questions.

DRUGS USED TO TREAT DISORDERS OF THE MIND OR PSYCHE

Major tranquillizers (antipsychotic/neuroleptic drugs)

The group of drugs that has had perhaps the most significant effect on the treatment of psychiatric illness are the class of drugs variously referred to as ANTIPSYCHOTIC or NEUROLEPTIC drugs, or simply MAJOR TRANQUILLIZERS. These now form the mainstay of pharmacological therapy of *schizophrenia* and, along with psychological and social therapy, have brought about a situation in which many such patients can be 'treated' in the community with short periods of hospitalization for acute relapses, rather than it being necessary to confine them continuously in a protected, institutional environment.

Schizophrenia is a condition (or group of conditions) characterized by a disturbed relationship between the inner and outer world, which is diagnosed on the basis of characteristic behaviour patterns and reported experiences of the patient. Auditory hallucinations or 'voices' (in the absence of real external voices), delusions (often of a paranoid or bizarre nature, with a twisted perspective on genuine events and no capacity for responding to reason), abnormal thought processes, and disturbed inter-personal relationships, are among the most common symptoms.

Three diagnostic criteria, *hallucinations*, *delusions* and *abnormal thought processes* are the prime features of a *psychosis*. Acute psychotic episodes can occur as an effect (side-effect) of certain drugs, or as a result of shattering personal experience such as a sudden bereavement, or in association with a severe clinical depression. However, the most likely diagnosis in a case of chronic psychosis is schizophrenia.

Before the advent of neuroleptic (antipsychotic) drugs in the early 1950s, treatment for such patients often consisted of isolation in a mental institution. Because of the nature of schizophrenia (i.e. disordered reasoning and logic) such patients were often out of reach of effective *psychotherapy*. Indeed one of the major advances that has come with pharmacological control of psychoses, is the much more useful interaction that it allows between the patient and those caring for them. Placing the achievements of antipsychotic drugs in perspective, one might say that there is clear evidence that they can shorten the duration of an acute psychotic episode and increase the time interval between relapses. By greatly reducing some of the *'positive'* symptoms of schizophrenia (i.e. violent/aggressive/inappropriate behaviour and hallucinations) they allow the possibility of psychotherapy, and make it possible for the patient to regain some sort of relationship with loved ones and friends, and generally live a more 'normal' life.

However, even the optimist would stop short of suggesting that antipsychotic drugs are in any sense a cure for the condition. More often than not, relapses will take place even while still taking these drugs (though these will be at longer time intervals). It is also true that delusions and *'negative'* symptoms (e.g. apathy, withdrawal and lack of verbal communication) are generally less successfully treated by the major tranquillizers than are the positive symptoms. The other major deficiency of neuroleptic drugs is that they can produce many side-effects, some serious. Apart from the high degree of sedation many tend to produce, perhaps the most serious side-effects are the disorders of motor/muscle control such as *dystonias* (continual or intermittent contraction of individual muscle groups), a 'restless-legs syndrome' (*akathisia*), Parkinsonian-like effects (slow movements, cog-wheel rigidity and tremor) and, perhaps most worrying of all, *tardive dyskinesias* – which unlike the first three may not be reversible on ceasing the drug, nor treatable by further drugs. Stereotypic, repetitive movements of the hand and wrist ('pill rolling') and of the lips, tongue, and jaw are the most common signs of tardive dyskinesias. The first three motor side-effects occur within days or weeks of starting treatment and may then decline with continuing therapy, but the latter may not appear until years of treatment have gone by (hence the term tardive), and by this time they may not resolve on stopping the drug.

Major tranquillizers, antipsychotic or neuroleptic drugs have for many years been a very important element in the treatment of psychotic patients. As can be seen from the points discussed above, the benefits and limitations of such therapy need to be clearly understood by family members and carers as well as the professionals responsible for their treatment. The reader might like to refer to some entries in the A to Z to gain some idea of the overall properties of these drugs, which are quite diverse in their chemical and pharmacological characteristics: e.g. CHLORPROMAZINE, FLUPENTHIXOL, HALOPERIDOL, CLOZAPINE.

Minor tranquillizers (anxiolytic, sedative, hypnotic actions)
Following on from discussion of the MAJOR TRANQUILLIZERS, the other group of drugs that have been described as tranquillizers are the MINOR TRANQUILLIZERS. These are quite different in effect, mechanism of action and usage to the major tranquillizers. They have three principal uses; as HYPNOTICS (drugs to help people sleep), as SEDATIVES (to calm individuals in an acute state of agitation over, for example, a bereavement), and as ANXIOLYTICS (drugs to treat people with anxiety states). By far the most important group of drugs of this type are the BENZODIAZEPINES.

These drugs had been used in therapy for many years before their mechanism of action was uncovered. They work by increasing the action of the inhibitory neurotransmitter called *gamma-aminobutyric acid* (*GABA*). It seems quite appropriate that an increase in inhibition of certain parts of the brain should have a calming or sleep-promoting effect. Indeed, if the reverse occurs, and the production or action of GABA is completely reduced by drugs, then convulsions result. Even more interestingly, some recently synthesised, atypical benzodiazepines, with the capacity to reduce rather than to increase the action of GABA, have been reported to cause terrifying anxiety attacks.

The potential usefulness of the benzodiazepines was first recognised in studies in animals where the drugs were shown to produce a calming effect. The drugs quickly established themselves in clinical practice in humans, and became the most popular anxiolytic/hypnotic agents used. Apart from being highly effective, they had major advantages over the other main group of drugs then used for these purposes, namely the BARBITURATES. Benzodiazepines proved to be less toxic in normal use, and much less dangerous in overdose (whether accidental or deliberate). At the outset it was also apparent that they were not as addictive as barbiturates – which by that time had become notable drugs of addiction (*habituation*) through over-use. With the passage of time, however, it has become recognised that benzodiazepines, particularly the short-acting type, can with prolonged use also create a powerful addiction. In such cases, attempts to stop drug treatment may produce such a strong *withdrawal syndrome* that reinstatement of drug prescription may be necessary. There have also been isolated reports that long-term use of some benzodiazepines may lead to psychotic symptoms with paranoia; further there are some indications that these drugs, although they seem to 'tranquillize' subjects, may not actually decrease the subjects' level of aggression. These are worrying findings, but it should not be thought that the benzodiazepines are necessarily dangerous or ineffective agents. Used responsibly, and ideally for short periods of time (i.e. days rather than weeks or months), these drugs are valuable and reliable additions to the medical armoury of the general practitioner, the hospital doctor and the psychiatrist. Examples of typical benzodiazepines include: **long-acting hypnotics**, NITRAZEPAM, FLUNITRAZEPAM, FLURAZEPAM; **short-acting hypnotics**, LOPRAZOLAM, LORMETAZEPAM, TENAZEPAM, TRIAZOLAM; **long-acting anxiolytics**; DIAZEPAM,

ALPRAZOLAM, BROMAZEPAM, CHLORDIAZEPOXIDE, CLORAZEPATE, MEDAZEPAM; **shorter-acting anxiolytics**, LORAZEPAM, OXAZEPAM. It should be noted that a number of other drug classes are also used for their hypnotic and anxiolytic actions.

Depression and antidepressant drugs

Disorders in which depression is a major component fall into two main groups, *bipolar disorder*, often called *manic-depression*, and simple or *unipolar depression*. The latter type will be discussed first in this section.

Some texts refer to clinical depression as an *affective disorder* (affect in this case means mood), others classify it as a *neurosis*. The latter is frequently used to describe psychiatric conditions where the problem, be it slight or severe, can be described as an extension or amplification of feelings or behaviour that most individuals occasionally suffer from, but which are normally of short duration or low intensity. This is distinct from a *psychosis* where the processes of thought and perception are distorted and outside normal experience. Depression, severe chronic anxiety and severe claustrophobia might well be termed neuroses. Clinical depression therefore, is reasonably straightforward to describe by reference to everyone's experience of suffering periods of depressed mood. Thus, symptoms such as lack of self-esteem, feelings of hopelessness or even suicidal thoughts, failure to derive pleasure from anything, lack of motivation, lack of energy, restlessness, lack of concentration, poor sleeping habits, preoccupation with physical ailments true or imagined, altered eating patterns, guilt, etc. are common in depression. When several of these symptoms occur in concert and are severe enough to obstruct an individual's capacity to function at work and at home, and when such incapacitation is persistent, then the individual may be said to be clinically depressed. Among such individuals one can recognise different subgroups of unipolar depression.

Major depression with *melancholia* is self-explanatory and is perhaps the most common subgroup. Much less common is major depression with *psychotic symptoms*, in which delusions and even hallucinations may be present. Among patients with depression, some display a definite *seasonal* pattern with, for example, periods of severe depression peaking in late autumn, and being least in the bright days of spring and mid-summer. Less severe forms of depression are often classified as *dysthymia*.

Perhaps more than any other psychiatric condition, depression has attracted a number of theories as to specific neurotransmitter disturbances which might account for, or at least be present in depression. For the most part such theories have been based on the effects of drugs with defined effects on brain chemistry. For instance the first and still the most widely prescribed classes of antidepressants are the MONOAMINE-OXIDASE INHIBITORS (MAOIS) and the TRICYCLIC ANTIDEPRESSANTS. These have the capacity to increase the level of neurotransmitter at those synapses where either *noradrenaline* or *serotonin* are neurotransmitters. (This and other findings led to the so-called amine theory of depression.) However, there is doubt about the true mechanism of action, in that although the effect on neurotransmitter amines happens within hours of starting the treatment, the beneficial effects (of the tricyclic antidepressants in particular) are not seen for nearly two weeks. Thus, it may be an adaptive response to the continued presence of the drugs that is, in fact, responsible for their primary beneficial effect. In view of these uncertainties it seems still too early to make any confident claims as to how these drugs actually act in the treatment of depression.

Many depressed patients respond very well to tricyclic antidepressants with an individual showing improved responsiveness and heightened levels of social interaction after about two weeks treatment with the drug. This may then provide the first opportunity for *psychotherapy* to be attempted and a combination of the two treatments is often valuable. In the event of the tricyclic antidepressants being ineffective and there being no possibility that the drug dosage, for one reason or another, is not reaching adequate levels in the blood, then it would be reasonable to consider the use of the monoamine oxidase inhibitors. These agents, however, have a lower success rate overall in the treatment of depression, and can only be used in patients with the capacity to comply with the dietary restrictions necessary to prevent the potentially fatal episodes of high blood pressure (the so-called 'cheese reaction'), which can be evoked by some common foods in patients taking these drugs. This reaction is due to the presence of SYMPATHOMIMETIC amines (e.g. *tyramine*) in certain foodstuffs; and patients may be given a printed card advising them against this risk (of eating food including cheese, pickled herrings, broad-bean pods, Bovril, Oxo, Marmite, 'high' game; or taking certain medicines particularly treatments for coughs and colds, tonics, etc.).

In the event of a severe depression not being relieved by treatment with either tricyclic or MAOI drugs, then controlled electro-convulsive therapy (ECT) would be considered. Despite its rather poor public image, it remains the most rapidly acting and perhaps successful treatment available.

Manic-depressive illness (bipolar disorder)
The characteristic pattern of this illness is one of periods of normality punctuated by episodes of *mania* and bouts of depression. Because of these mood swings around the norm the disorder is sometimes called *bipolar disorder*. The depressions are similar to those seen in major unipolar depression, discussed above; while the term mania is used to describe a mood disorder in which the level of mental and motor activity is greatly heightened. Speech and ideas seem to rush into and through the patient's consciousness in a breathless dash. Sleep and relaxation are much reduced but patients seem to able to keep going with limitless energy and, though the mood can sometimes be euphoric, it is more commonly restless and impatient. Social judgement is severely impaired and the activities of manic patients are, at the least, wearing on carers. Sexual promiscuity, uncontrolled spending sprees and alcohol and drug abuse are not uncommon in some manic patients. *Psychotic symptoms* can be present, most frequently in the form of grandiose delusions of power. When these mood swings either side of normality are recurring, but consistently of lesser severity, the condition may be termed *cyclothymia*. A notable advance in our approach to understanding manic depressive illness is the realization that in some cases there is a strong familial (i.e. hereditary) factor, which can be localized to a particular gene (on the 11th chromosome). If the function of this gene and associated factors can be probed, then we may truly be near to understanding an important element in the puzzle of manic-depressive illness.

In manic-depressive illness it is often a manic phase that presents the acute need for treatment and initially ANTIPSYCHOTIC drugs (major tranquillizers) will be prescribed. These should reduce the mania within 24 hours and then maintenance therapy with a distinctly different psychoactive agent, LITHIUM, may be gradually instituted in suitable patients. The apparently highly specific beneficial effect of lithium (which is a metallic element, usually given by mouth as lithium carbonate or citrate salts), as a drug in the treatment of manic-depressive illness, was first noticed some 30 years ago; and after a long period establishing safe ways to control its dosage, it has now become the dominant agent in the treatment of this condition. Following the achievement of a satisfactory level of lithium in the bloodstream (measured chemically in blood samples taken at regular intervals), the antipsychotic therapy (i.e. the major tranquillizer, not the lithium) may be discontinued, though it should be reinstated if psychotic symptoms recur. In addition to the drug therapy, psychotherapy and family or group support therapy may be very useful in preventing or ameliorating violent mood swings. Although lithium is a very useful drug it is not without side-effects. Nausea, vomiting and diarrhoea may be troublesome though they usually lessen with continued treatment. Also, tremor and thirst are recognised early side-effects, which may recede with time. Lithium may also cause a reduction in the production of thyroid hormone, a side-effect which itself may require drug treatment. Such side-effects certainly increase with dose and it is prudent to keep the dose to the minimum and be prepared to use other specialist agents for major mood swings.

While lithium alone may reduce the occurrence and severity of manic episodes in manic-depressive illness, the occurrence of a severe episode of depression usually requires treatment with a TRICYCLIC ANTIDEPRESSANT drug (see above), and this class of drug can often prove very successful in this situation.

DRUGS USED TO TREAT PAIN – ANALGESICS

The protective function of pain

Pain is an unpleasant, but vital, sensation. Its function is to warn us that the affected part of the body is damaged or under stress. Without pain, damage can proceed unheeded and unchecked. The rare children who are born without the capacity to feel pain inevitably suffer severe damage to vulnerable areas such as tongues, lips, toes, and fingers, to the extent of causing permanent deformities. Worse, they may be subject to life-threatening traumas, such as a fractured limb or ruptured appendix, without realising the emergency. In the evolutionary context, therefore, pain is an invaluable sense in the preservation of a state of well-being. To the individual, however, pain, particularly when it seems purely 'destructive', can constitute a terrible burden. Thus for the patient with severe rheumatoid arthritis or some types of cancer, pain may be severe and ever-present. To know that the pain is caused by tissue damage at a particular site is of little value if the condition responds poorly to treatment.

Drugs used to suppress the sensation of pain are called ANALGESICS, or 'pain-killers' in popular terminology. To understand the way in which analgesics work, it is worth examining the pathway of pain messages from injured tissue to brain.

1. At the source of the pain signal the small sensory nerve endings that carry the pain message are activated by a stimulus such as pressure, heat, stretch, or chemicals released from inflamed tissues or directly introduced into the tissues (e.g. a wasp sting).

2. The electrical signals generated by these stimuli travel in the nerves to the spinal cord, and there initiate electrical signals in a second nerve trunk, which ascends into the brain itself.

3. Then from within the brain, the pain signals do three things:
   a) they disseminate general activating-signals that put the brain on the alert.
   b) they provide specific localising information to indicate the source of the pain.
   c) they give rise to the unpleasant subjective sensation that we describe as 'pain'.

Narcotic and non-narcotic analgesics

Analgesics fall into two general classes. The first group of drugs, many very powerful, are the narcotic analgesics: these are related pharmacologically, and generally chemically, to MORPHINE (found along with opium and other compounds, in the seed-head of the opium poppy (*Papaver somniferum*). They were originally termed narcotics since they can produce a state of *narcosis* (see discussion below), but this meaning is effectively lost today – since the term has become synonymous with 'illegal' drugs (at least in the USA). This class of drugs, including morphine, PETHIDINE, CODEINE, and DIAMORPHINE *(heroin),* are more usefully called OPIATES (pharmacologically and chemically like opium or morphine) or OPIOIDS (pharmacologically like both morphine and the natural endogenous peptide mediators of the brain, e.g. the ENKEPHALINS).

The second group, the non-narcotic analgesics, include drugs like ASPIRIN, PARACETAMOL and IBUPROFEN. These do not produce narcosis, and some are widely used against inflammatory states like rheumatoid arthritis.

Both classes of pain-killing drugs are invaluable, but for different applications. Experience has taught that the aspirin-like drugs are useful for sprains, bruises, toothache, and mild rheumatic conditions. For more severe pain, such as serious tissue injury, or a heart attack, or acute post-operative pain following major surgery, or some cases of terminal cancer, the aspirin-like drugs are often ineffective and narcotic analgesics like morphine are the only agents that can provide relief.

What is it then that so separates these two types of analgesic? Some 20 years ago one might have been fairly confident in claiming that for the most part the non-narcotic analgesics, such as aspirin, acted purely at the site of the tissue injury to prevent the formation and release of chemicals, called prostaglandins, which normally enhance the genesis of pain signals in the pain-carrying sensory nerve-endings of the affected tissue. Thus they appeared to act by depressing an important component of the inflammatory response causing the pain. This action of drugs, such as aspirin and ibuprofen, is similar to that of steroids such as hydrocortisone (so they are often referred to as NON-STEROIDAL ANTI-INFLAMMATORY drugs (NSAIDS). To ascribe the analgesic action of such drugs to their anti-inflammatory action seemed a natural progression of ideas. However, this simple concept was challenged at an early stage by the properties of paracetamol, which is an effective non-narcotic analgesic – but has very little anti-inflammatory effect. This dilemma still remains to be settled, and there are now many drugs of the non-narcotic analgesic class for which it is recognised that their analgesic activity does not go hand in hand with their anti-inflammatory action. It would seem likely that their additional analgesic action is exerted at some other site, perhaps within the brain, but even this is not certain.

In contrast to the relatively recent history of the NSAIDS, opium compounds from the ripe seed-head of the opium poppy have been highly prized for thousands of years for their ability to 'transport' the subject, albeit temporarily, to 'another world' where pain and suffering seem much more distant. Also by way of contrast with the NSAIDS, the narcotic analgesics can exert a very powerful analgesic action. The term narcotic arises out of the capacity of these drugs to induce a state of complete sedation or 'sleep' (*narkosis* – Greek for 'state of numbness') with high doses. Unfortunately if too much of the drug is administered or taken accidentally, then this state can very readily slip into one of coma and complete respiratory depression (i.e. cessation of breathing leading to death).

The narcotic analgesics depress the brain's appreciation of painful events by actions at several levels within the central nervous system. First, they depress the transmission of pain signals from the peripheral sensory nerves at the level of the spinal cord, so reducing the signal going to the brain. Second, they depress the neuronal events stimulated by pain signals at the lower levels of the brain. Third, they alter the perception or recognition (cognition) of pain at higher centres within the brain, at the level of 'appreciation' with all that this entails. Thus, even though a treated individual may still be 'aware' of the pain, he or she will be less disturbed by it. The reassurance that severe pain can be controlled, even if further increases in dose are necessary, may be one of the most liberating aspects of analgesic therapy.

Unlike the NSAIDS, narcotic analgesics are apt to generate tolerance, necessitating a steady increase in dose to achieve the same degree of analgesia. This is undoubtedly linked to their potential for generating addiction (*habituation*). When the drugs are first taken, the body is immediately affected by these drugs – but almost as quickly it adapts to their presence in such a a way that their effect is lessened. On the second dose, more of the drug is needed to achieve the same effect in the 'adapted' individual, and so it goes on, with the body attempting all the time to counteract the increasing doses of the drug by increasing, in turn, its level of adaptation. If the drug is then withheld, the body is out of normal balance and, in the absence of the drug, its by now adapted behaviour is inappropriate, and a *withdrawal syndrome* is seen. This is often, not surprisingly, opposite in character to the effects produced by the drug. Thus, a craving for the drug, agitation, insomnia, sweating, tremor, griping pains in the stomach and intestines, runny nose and eyes, dilated pupils, aching limbs, nausea, vomiting, diarrhoea, fever, and elevated pulse-rate are among the unpleasant effects of withdrawal. When withdrawal is attempted after a long period of habituation to high doses, these effects may be almost intolerable and, as they can last for days, the craving to resort again to the drug can be unbearable. The unpleasantness of withdrawal coupled to the pleasurable effects of taking the drug, make the opioids perhaps the most addictive of all compounds known. History and literature in most cultures are full of accounts of the perils of addiction to preparations containing morphine-like narcotic analgesics, especially opium and laudanum (which is an alcoholic solution of opium).

These then, are the most familiar properties and actions of narcotic analgesics. What may not be so familiar are other effects which include: nausea (on the first few occasions of taking the drug); an ANTITUSSIVE effect (suppression of the cough reflex), which can be very useful in the treatment of persistent, unproductive coughing; and a profound constipating effect, which for some patients almost negates the beneficial effects. Indeed, patients treated with high doses of narcotic preparations should always be considered for parallel treatment with laxatives, though in other circumstances the ANTIDIARRHOEAL action of opiates may indeed be beneficial.

Improvements in opioid-like analgesics and their use

A massive research effort by pharmacologists and neuroscientists over the last 30 years has revealed that there are distinct differences (*sub-types*) in the *receptors* on neurones through which opioid-like analgesics bring about their various actions. These receptors are present on neurones within the central nervous system to 'recognise' the various *endogenous* (naturally present) opioid mediators within the brain. The demonstration of the existence of these 'natural analgesics' (which include the related peptide families called *enkephalins*, *dynorphins* and *endorphins*) has invigorated research into pain mechanisms, and has raised hopes that more specific analgesic drugs may be found, which can perhaps mimic the natural mediator at just one receptor sub-type or to a limited extent. Thus it may be possible to depress pain without, for example, producing addiction or depressing respiration or producing constipation. So far, however, this hope remains somewhat elusive, though there is now available a much greater range of opioid analgesics with a wide range of properties such as solubility, onset of effect, duration of action and maximum effect.

A perhaps more clinically significant development of recent years has been the increasing sophistication in the administration of narcotic analgesics. This is typified by the introduction of small continuous intravenous infusion pumps which, once set up, can allow much more convenient and flexible control by nursing staff or even patients themselves. The equipment involves some expense, and it certainly increases the tangle of 'tubes' attached to the patient, but it does mean that the level of analgesia can be readily maintained over an extended period and adjusted without the need to call a doctor or revisit the medicines cabinet. Once such a device is primed with an appropriate amount of analgesic solution, it can be set to deliver a constant volume per hour. This rate can be adjusted by the attendant nursing staff. In *PCA* (*patient-controlled-analgesia*), the patient (even children as young as five or six years) can increase or decrease the rate of administration, according to their subjective feelings of pain, by pressing a button on the device. An automatic 'lock-out' period, of say 15 minutes after each button press, prevents any risk of overdosing. With children in particular, this technique frees them from the fear of painful intramuscular injections with a needle and greatly improves their acceptance of pain control.

Analgesia in surgery and post-operative recovery
One might imagine that GENERAL ANAESTHESIA (absence of sensation) used in carrying out surgical procedures, would not require the addition of analgesia (suppression of pain), but in fact the two terms are neither linguistically nor scientifically synonymous. An effective dose of a long-acting analgesic (given as a premedication) may allow the use of a significantly lower level of general anaesthesia – and this may be much to the benefit of the patient. It will also provide analgesic 'cover' in the immediate post-operative period when the patient will be disturbed by pain, but may not be sufficiently coherent to indicate their level of awareness or request analgesics. Continuing analgesic cover for several more days may greatly ease the stress of post-operative recovery. Such cover may be provided by a narcotic analgesic given by intramuscular injections, or by intravenous infusions (controlled either by the patient or by the medical/nursing staff). Of course, in this situation one would not want to risk the danger of addiction, but as the pain arising out of the surgery decreases so does the need for strong analgesics. In many cases non-narcotic analgesics can usefully complement narcotic analgesics in providing analgesic cover.

Analgesics in care of the terminally ill patient
The treatment of terminally ill patients (commonly from cancer), is an area in which narcotic opiate analgesics have proved invaluable. Of course, not all individuals with cancer suffer severe pain, but for those who do, opiates provide the most acceptable all-round solution. In this situation the problem of addiction is not a

cause for concern and tolerance, which will inevitably develop, can be overcome by increasing the dose. Constipation will remain as a drawback to the use of these drugs, though awareness of the problem and concurrent laxative treatment will usually prove successful. *Patient-controlled-analgesia* (PCA) can provide great reassurance to the patient and remove some of the strain on untrained helpers in trying to decide when the next dose of analgesic should be given. Undoubtedly, to prevent the breakthrough of severe pain, large doses of narcotic analgesic will be necessary and this will result in a significant degree of sedation. At least in PCA the balance between two evils, pain and unacceptable sedation, can be struck by patients themselves. It is perhaps in the hospice movement that the importance of good pain control in the terminally ill patient has been most appreciated. Ultimately, as bodily systems fail, it may be that analgesics, by depressing vital centres for respiration and blood pressure, hasten the end, but to many this may seem a welcome release.

Analgesia in childbirth

The majority of women in this country today are glad of the option of some degree of pain relief during childbirth. Pain experienced in the process of labour and the actual birth is of course perceived by many women as somehow different to that of disease, but were such pain to be experienced by the average male it would, one suspects, be graded severe. Controlled relaxation and deep breathing can achieve some ameliorating effect, but for the majority of women analgesic cover is most welcome. There are problems however. If an agent is to be administered to the mother how can it be prevented from having an undesirable effect on the baby both *in utero* and after birth? If the mother is to be relieved of painful stimuli from the uterus and birth canal area, will it diminish her capacity to 'push' and give birth? How will analgesic procedures, even if they are desired, affect the mother's feelings about such a personal event?

For some years now the standard analgesic techniques employed in British obstetric wards have been: 'gas and air' mixtures (actually nitrous oxide gas – as analgesic – mixed with pure oxygen in roughly equal proportions); PETHIDINE, the narcotic analgesic, by intramuscular injection; or LOCAL ANAESTHETIC analgesia by epidural injection.

The first technique, nitrous oxide/oxygen mixture, is readily administered and safe (in that their depressant effects are slight and both the new born baby and the mother will rapidly 'blow off' the nitrous oxide). However, for many women the level of analgesia actually achieved is found to be insufficient.

The second technique, intramuscular pethidine, is not nearly as controllable or flexible, but it can produce a much greater degree of analgesia. However the drug, as well as affecting the mother, readily enters the unborn baby's circulation resulting in analgesia and some degree of vital function depression at birth. However, this depression is rarely serious, and if necessary a rapidly-acting opiate antagonist can be administered to the new-born baby to nullify the effects of any pethidine in its circulation.

The third, epidural local anaesthetic analgesia (see also under this heading below) is more 'high-tech' and certainly more *invasive*, but it is controllable, and can extend the clinical options if surgical assistance is called for in a hurry. The technique depends upon injecting a local anaesthetic into the epidural space that surrounds the nerve trunks as they enter or leave the spinal cord. The anaesthetic diffuses into the nerve fibres, blocking their conduction of impulses, including those carrying the pain signals. The baby is unaffected, and with careful placement of the injection the degree of impairment of functions other than lower abdominal/perineal sensation and motor control of the legs should be slight. In the hands of experienced staff the procedure is very safe and midwives may be trained to administer the injections (though may not put the injection needle in position). In a recent development, opioid analgesics have been given by the same epidural route and found to be produce some analgesic effect. It seems likely that a combination of opioid and local anaesthetic by the epidural route may soon be used in some centres.

Choice of analgesic

As outlined above, the severity and type of pain being treated largely determines whether narcotic or non-narcotic analgesics are used. The treatment of rheumatic conditions is largely outside the scope of this book (though most NSAIDS in use for such states are included in the A to Z section for completeness), but it may be noted that the most suitable drug for a particular patient (e.g. NAPROXEN, INDOMETHACIN, MEFENAMIC ACID, PIROXICAM or SUNDILAC), is arrived at partly by trial and entails consideration of the severity of the side-effects in relation to clinical benefit. In choosing over-the-counter analgesics however, legislation sensibly allows no drugs with marked side-effects to be sold to the public. This reduces the selection to ASPIRIN, IBUPROFEN, PARACETAMOL, and CODEINE (the latter in combination). Of these, paracetamol is a safe drug (except in overdose) and is suitable for fevers and minor pains and headaches – but lacks anti-inflammatory activity so is of less use where the pain is related to tissue damage. Aspirin and ibuprofen are better in the latter case, but there may be gastrointestinal disturbance. Codeine is a narcotic analgesic so it is not available alone for self-medication, but it is available at low dose in combination with one or other of the other analgesics mentioned. Some mixed analgesic preparations contain CAFFEINE, but this is of unproven value (though it may provide some 'lift' when the subject feels low), and is not recommended combined with aspirin since it may well increase gastric erosion. Details of some over-the-counter compound preparations may be found in the A to Z section under CO-CODAMOL and CO-CODAPRIN as well as under individual names. It should be noted that proprietary preparations are often considerably more expensive than their generic equivalents, but offer no real advantages.

DRUGS USED TO TREAT NEUROLOGICAL DISORDERS OF THE BRAIN

Epilepsy and anti-epileptic drugs

In epilepsy there are episodes of involuntary, unpremeditated activity in specific brain-circuits, which produce characteristic signs and symptoms dependent on the particular circuits involved. Thus for example, if there is involuntary firing of brain-circuits controlling the nerves to the facial and jaw muscles, then whenever an epileptic event (*seizure*) occurs there may be involuntary twitching of the mouth. More dramatically, in the condition known by the term *Grand Mal* (*tonic-clonic seizures*), a seizure involves an initial *'aura'* with perhaps a feeling of impending unpleasantness, followed rapidly by unconsciousness, and powerful and sustained (*tonic*) extension of the limbs. The individual, if standing, falls to the ground and within a minute or so the rigidity of the limbs gives way to rhythmic jerking (*clonic*) movements that gradually subside, leaving the individual in a comatose state, which in turn passes into sleep from which awakening takes place. The individual will usually have no recollection of events over a time-period starting just before the seizure.

In a form of epilepsy more common in children, called *Petit Mal* or *absence seizures*, there is much less disturbance of muscle function. Indeed the child will not usually lose posture, and the only clear sign that something is amiss may be a few seconds' loss of attention. However, whereas in many cases of Grand Mal, the seizures are relatively infrequent, in contrast, in Petit Mal there may be hundreds of seizures in a single week. Happily, Petit Mal often recedes at the age of puberty.

Another type of epilepsy that should be mentioned is *Temporal Lobe Epilepsy* (a type of partial epilepsy sometimes called *Psychomotor epilepsy*). Here the *focus* of the disorder is thought to reside in the temporal lobe of the cerebral hemispheres. This part of the brain is involved in complex integration of sensory, motor, cognitive and emotional aspects of brain function. The seizures are therefore often correspondingly complex in form, perhaps producing outbursts of erratic behaviour – such as sudden incoherent speech patterns or complex, involuntary patterns of motor activity such as wringing of the hands. This form of epilepsy often produces disturbing patterns of amnesia and episodes of depression (probably in response to the condition, rather than a feature of the condition itself).

In many epileptic individuals, epilepsy is the only sign of imperfect function of the brain, and there is every prospect in such individuals that drug treatment will control the seizures, allowing them to lead a perfectly normal life. However, there are others in whom epilepsy is but one of a number of indicators of significant brain damage and in these cases the seizures may be more unresponsive to drug therapy.

The drugs used to treat epilepsy may differ, depending on the type of epilepsy being treated. Thus *tonic-clonic* and *partial* (*focal*) *seizures* (involving primarily the cerebral cortex) are best treated by one group of drugs (e.g. CARBAMAZEPINE, PHENYTOIN, PHENOBARBITONE); while a different group (e.g. ETHOSUXIMIDE) is used to treat *absence seizures* where the focus of the disorder is thought to lie deeper in the brain. Yet another group of drugs has wide-spectrum anti-epileptic activity and may be used to treat many different types of epilepsy (e.g. SODIUM VALPROATE).

As in all other situations in which drugs are to be administered over a long period of time (an epileptic individual may require life-time treatment) there may be problems with side-effects. Drowsiness, depression of intellectual performance, and disturbances of balance are perhaps the most frequently encountered problems. The optimal dose for each individual should be arrived at by a process of balancing suppression of epileptic phenomena against acceptability or otherwise of side-effects. Pregnancy may raise difficulties as some of the drugs of this class are known to increase, albeit slightly, the risk of teratogenic effects (damage to the unborn child). With all anti-epileptic drugs it is important to remember to take the drugs at the prescribed intervals, because missing the drugs for a few days brings on what is in effect a withdrawal state when the likelihood of seizures is raised above normal. However, one might also want to withdraw the drug altogether if the individual has been seizure-free for a number of years. This introduces a dilemma, for if a seizure does occur in this vulnerable period it may mean the individual will lose the hard-won privilege of a valid driving licence, because this requires a seizure-free period. Despite these cautionary remarks, anti-epileptic treatments can be judged a success and highly beneficial for many epileptics.

Parkinson's disease and antiparkinsonian drugs

Parkinson's disease is almost unique among disorders of the brain, in that the principal defect is clearly established, and consequently a rational strategy of drug treatment is now possible. In this degenerative condition there is an accelerated rate of loss of pigmented neurones in a discrete cluster (a *nucleus*) at the base of the brain called the *substantia nigra* (black body). The processes from the nerve cells in this nucleus ascend to a area higher in the brain called the *striatum*. This lies underneath the cerebral cortex and is involved in the programming and control of movement. The neurones from the substantia nigra release a *neurotransmitter* called *dopamine* onto neurones in the striatum. In Parkinson's disease, because of the loss of the cells releasing dopamine, one sees the characteristic features of this disease, namely: slowness of movement, 'cogwheel'-type rigidity, and resting tremor. Difficulty in initiating movement, poverty of facial expression, drooling and difficulties with speech and swallowing, may also be present. The condition is progressive but variable in rate of progression.

Current drug therapy for Parkinson's disease is based upon two basic ideas about *neurotransmitter imbalance* in this condition.

1. there is a deficiency of release of the neurotransmitter dopamine in the striatum.

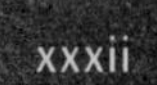

2. this produces a consequent exaggeration of the influence of the neurotransmitter acetylcholine in the striatum.

In historical terms the second point was recognised first, largely because drugs inhibiting the action of the neurotransmitter acetylcholine (ANTICHOLINERGIC drugs) were found (empirically) to ameliorate some of the symptoms of Parkinson's disease, notably the tremor and the excessive salivation. Once the critical deficiency of dopamine was discovered, attention switched to replacing or restoring the dopamine deficiency. The first and still most satisfactory approach was to administer L-DOPA (LEVODOPA), the natural chemical precursor of dopamine. When this enters the brain, it is taken up by the remaining dopaminergic nerve terminals in the striatum, converted to dopamine, and released from these nerves at a higher-than-normal rate; so restoring the balance. Such an approach is obviously limited by the number of dopaminergic neurones still remaining, and ultimately, when all these neurones degenerate, this drug would be expected to become ineffective.

In a sophistication of this approach, an additional drug (e.g. CARBIDOPA or BENSERAZIDE) was added to the levodopa preparation to inhibit the utilization of the latter outside the brain, thereby reducing the oral dose required and also limiting some of the side-effects. In more recent developments other drugs have been tried with some success. These include drugs that mimic the action of dopamine itself (e.g. BROMOCRIPTINE, LYSURIDE), and those that inhibit the inactivation of dopamine. This latter group of drugs include ones (e.g. SELEGILINE) that prevent the breakdown of dopamine by specific enzymes, and there is a slight possibility (as yet not convincingly demonstrated in terms of clinical trials) that they may be able to arrest the rate of progression of the underlying pathology in Parkinson's disease.

Almost inevitably these various drug treatments for Parkinson's disease have side-effects. The inevitability arises out of the fact that the transmitters that are either inhibited or restored by these treatments have important roles outside the specific sites involved in Parkinsonian pathology. Thus dopamine is involved in hormonal control mechanisms, mood-control and thought processes, as well as movement control. All of these are likely to be affected with levodopa treatment though usually not to any great degree. The anticholinergic antiparkinsonian agents (e.g. BENZHEXOL) will typically produce sedation, dry mouth, constipation, difficulties in micturition (urination) and effects on focusing of the eyes. There is no doubt, however, that drug treatment can greatly improve the lot of the Parkinson's disease sufferer.

Lest confusion arise, a clear distinction must be made between the descriptions of the side-effects of drugs used to treat a patient who has Parkinson's disease, and the side-effects that are commonly referred to as *parkinsonian-like* (or *extrapyramidal*), which may arise from the use of quite different drugs for other purposes. The most common examples lie with the MAJOR TRANQUILLIZER or ANTIPSYCHOTIC drugs (as discussed above) (e.g. FLUPHENAZINE, HALOPERIDOL).

Interestingly, a chemical called MPTP, which came to prominence in the USA as an impurity in an illegally synthesised preparation of a well-known drug of abuse, was first picked up because 'users' of that batch of drug were turning up with classic signs of severe Parkinson's disease although they were atypically young to be suffering that condition. Investigation of the nature of the toxic action of this chemical is, paradoxically, now proving extremely valuable in research into the cause and treatment of the 'natural' form of Parkinson's disease.

Alzheimer's disease and prospective drug therapies

Alzheimer's disease is a disorder of the brain characterized, in behavioural terms, by progressive *dementia* affecting particularly learning and memory in the early stages of the condition. In neurochemical terms, the characteristic features are abnormal aggregations of material in the brain called *neurofibrillary tangles* and *senile plaques*. A major chemical constituent of the latter is an abnormal and highly insoluble peptide of the so-called *amyloid* type (presumably created by abnormal processing of a normal body peptide). Some cases of Alzheimer's disease (*familial Alzheimer's disease*) have been shown to have a hereditary basis, which is associated with a particular gene defect (on chromosome 21) thus pointing to a possible biochemical basis for the disorder. Current research is strongly directed towards discovering the cause of the disease. In the meantime new treatments continue to be tried, but in all truth none with any really significant effect has yet been demonstrated. Most treatments have been based on the early finding that a consistent neurochemical deficit in Alzheimer's is of neurones in the frontal cortices of the brain, which use the neurotransmitter *acetylcholine*. In a way analogous to the treatment of Parkinson's disease, attempts have been made to restore activity of the deficient system by replacing, or increasing synthesis, of the deficient natural acetylcholine, (e.g. by acetylcarnitine or by CHOLINE analogues), or decreasing its breakdown (e.g. ANTICHOLINESTERASES; tacrine hydrochloride).

Another neurotransmitter likely to be involved in memory processes is glutamate, and some therapeutic measures have attempted to modulate its neurochemistry and action, but so far without success in treating either the memory and cognitive defects in Alzheimer's disease.

In relation to possible causes of Alzheimer's disease, one might mention that excessive build-up of aluminium in the brain has been implicated as the cause of a similar type of dementia, which occurred in a few kidney-dialysis patients in the early days of the technique. Removal of high levels of aluminium from the dialysis fluid prevented the condition. This stimulated neuropathologists to look at post-mortem aluminium levels in the brains of Alzheimer patients. At first it was reported that very high levels were present in the plaques which are such a feature of the condition. In more recent studies it appears that only some Alzheimer patients have high aluminium levels in the plaques. Nevertheless it is an interesting observation. However, no very convincing evidence of a causative role for aluminium has come from studies of individuals exposed to high levels in the diet or by way of aluminium silicate antacid therapy.

There may be some justification in regarding Alzheimer's disease as one aspect of a wider problem of *age-associated memory impairment (AAMI)* and other memory defects. Here, there are those that believe drugs that increase blood supply to the brain (by dilating cerebral blood vessels, e.g. HYDERGINE) may be of value, but this remains to be proved. Yet others, by a step of reverse logic, hold that these and other drugs ('smart drugs') may enhance memory in normal individuals, and here only time will tell as to whether any such approach is possible (or safe).

DRUGS USED IN THE TREATMENT OF MISCELLANEOUS DISORDERS OF THE BRAIN

Migraine and anti-migraine drugs

Migraine is usually classified as either *'common'* or *'classical'*. In common migraine the main symptom is headache, either one- or both-sided, sometimes with feelings of nausea and, less commonly, actual vomiting. Drowsiness is common. Loud noises and bright light exacerbate the condition and most sufferers need to retire to a quiet dark place until the attack wanes. The length of an attack is generally measured in terms of hours and half-days. In *classical migraine*, in addition to the headache, *photophobia* (increased sensitivity to light) and nausea of *common migraine*, there are more prominent signs of neurological disturbance, often of the visual system, with flashing lights and even some sight loss.

Migraine attacks are often brought on by characteristic triggers such as stress or winding down from a period of sustained stress, and dietary factors (typically, cheese, caffeine, chocolate or citrus fruits, alcoholic drinks, or an extended interval between meals). For each individual the triggers have to be recognised and avoided. Despite intensive research it is not clear how these factors can initiate an attack. Indeed, there is still uncertainty over what is responsible for the headache and other symptoms. One major theory says it is a disturbance of neurones in the brain (*neurogenic hypothesis*), while another ascribes the symptoms to a disturbance of the blood vessels supplying the brain and cranium (*vascular hypothesis*). Both may be correct, in that the condition may have both neural and vascular components. If a neurotransmitter is involved in migraine, then *serotonin* (*5-hydroxytryptamine*) would be the preferred candidate. A certain chemical compound (*M-chlorophenylpiperazine*), which can mimic some of the actions of 5-HT, has been reported to provoke migraine attacks in a high proportion of migraine sufferers; also, other agents that release serotonin or block its uptake, may stimulate attacks.

Despite our very incomplete understanding of migraine, there seems reasonable agreement that relaxation of the muscular walls of the blood vessels (*vasodilatation*) supplying the cranium can cause headaches. Drugs that can restore a normal level of constriction to these blood vessels prevent such headaches. This evidence is strongly supportive of a vascular component to migraine headaches.

The treatment of migraine should be considered in terms of three distinct steps. First, identify and avoid precipitating factors. Second, treat acute attacks with ANALGESICS (to ameliorate the headache pain), ANTI-EMETICS (drugs to reduce nausea), and specific ANTI-MIGRAINE drugs. Third, if attacks are frequent and severe, consider *prophylactic drug treatment* (i.e. advance treatment to prevent or reduce the incidence of attacks). Analgesic and anti-emetic drugs are considered elsewhere in this Introduction.

The most widely prescribed specific anti-migraine drug is ERGOTAMINE, which constricts the cerebral and cranial blood vessels, and thereby improves the headache, though it does not benefit the other symptoms, i.e. visual disturbances and nausea. In the near-future a new anti-migraine drug, SUMATRIPTAN, is expected to be available and confirm promising reports from clinical trials. This drug, which can activate a discrete serotonin receptor subtype and constrict the cranial arteries, appears to reduce headaches significantly in about two-thirds of patients. Unlike ergotamine, it also appears to benefit the nausea and intolerance to light which accompany typical attacks.

For prophylactic treatment, the options are fairly wide, but the resulting effects are not usually outstanding and may not be sufficient to compensate for side-effects, or the risk thereof. Here, BETA-BLOCKERS, 5-HT (SEROTONIN) receptor blockers and calcium channel blockers are among the agents that have been tried.

Nausea and vomiting and anti-emetic drugs
There are three closely-related phenomena to consider under this heading: *vomiting* (otherwise known as *emesis*, i.e. the act of expulsion of the stomach contents); *retching* (which is generated by a similar but different pattern of activity in abdominal and respiratory muscles, but does not result in effective expulsion of stomach contents); and *nausea* (which is the sensation of feeling sick). The vomiting and retching reflexes involve highly complex patterns of muscle activity, which are coordinated by a brain centre called the medullary vomiting centre in the brain stem close to the respiratory centres. Apart from the sheer unpleasantness of these phenomena, which can cause extreme distress; vomiting, if persistent, causes the repeated loss of stomach contents, preventing adequate nourishment and leading to serious dehydration and imbalance of body electrolytes such as sodium, potassium and hydrogen ions. The patient will be weakened and may require intravenous 'feeding'. Drugs that can inhibit these phenomena are therefore very useful.

Clinically speaking, among the most common causes of severe nausea and vomiting are: *chemotherapy* with particular anti-cancer drugs (the worst drug in this respect being cisplatin); *radiotherapy* involving the upper-abdominal area; tumours; food poisoning; and blockages affecting the passage of food in the stomach and small intestine. A common factor in all of these stimuli, is the likelihood of increased sensory-nerve traffic coming from the stomach area. It is now known that both chemotherapy and abdominal radiation lead to the release of the substance called *serotonin* (*5-HT*) from cells in the gastrointestinal tract, and this mediator can chemically activate firing in the sensory nerves in that area through a stimulatory action on *serotonin* receptors of a specific subtype (5-HT_3): a finding that has promoted research into locating antagonists acting at this site (see ONDANSETRON, below).

Another notable cause of nausea and vomiting is *motion sickness*. Here the problem is due to disturbing, and possibly conflicting, information from various sensory systems such as the eyes and the *vestibular balance-centres* of the inner ear. Similar problems can arise in pathological disorders of the vestibular apparatus of the inner-ear (e.g. *Ménière's disease*). Pregnancy, of course, is the most common cause of nausea, but only in exceptional cases does it require anti-emetic treatment. Finally, another cause is chemical stimulation of what is called the *chemoreceptor trigger-zone* (in the *area postrema* of the brain medulla). This may be seen with OPIATE administration, or with centrally active analogues of the neurotransmitter *dopamine* (e.g. APOMORPHINE).

The early anti-emetics were of the ANTIHISTAMINE and ANTICHOLINERGIC classes. The former have a fairly wide application against many types of nausea, but the anticholinergics are largely used against *motion sickness* and other conditions disrupting balance centres. The next class of drug to arrive on the scene was the PHENOTHIAZINES, which have multiple pharmacological actions notably anticholinergic, antihistaminic and antidopaminergic properties. More recently, METOCLOPRAMIDE became the most widely prescribed anti-emetic for the treatment of vomiting caused by cancer chemotherapeutic agents. It was thought to work by preventing the action of the neurotransmitter dopamine in the chemoreceptor trigger-zone. Its ability to promote the normal passage of gastric contents into the duodenum may also be important. Because of its antidopaminergic actions it can cause side-effects; principally *dystonias* of the type seen with MAJOR TRANQUILLIZERS. The most recent anti-emetics to be recognised and introduced clinically are antagonists at the serotonin 5-HT_3 receptor subtype. ONDANSETRON is the first of this class to be marketed as such. Interestingly, at least some of its anti-emetic actions are likely to be by virtue of blocking the activation of sensory nerves in the gastrointestinal tract, which appear to cause the vomiting induced by chemotherapy. That is, its anti-emetic action is partly on the peripheral, rather than the central, nervous system.

DRUGS USED TO PRODUCE ANAESTHESIA

Anaesthesia means loss of sensation, and this may be achieved either by drugs that act only locally to the site of administration, the LOCAL ANAESTHETICS, or by agents that act on the brain to cause unconsciousness, the GENERAL ANAESTHETICS. As explained above in relation to the treatment of pain, this nomenclature tends to hide the purpose that lies behind the use of these drugs – which is generally to reduce the sensation of pain, commonly while some surgical or other manoeuvre takes place. For this reason, local anaesthetics may often also be referred to as local analgesics (particularly in the USA). In the case of the general anaesthetics, the loss of consciousness is almost incidental to their use. Because there is little connection between these two drug classes other than their type of use, they will be discussed separately.

Local anaesthetics

These may be applied at various sites, and in a number of ways, to block the transmission of information along nerves to the brain, including the sensory nerves that convey the painful stimuli. At the simplest level, a local anaesthetic cream (e.g. of AMETHOCAINE) may be applied to unbroken skin or mucous membranes, and some suitable preparations are available over the counter, and may well provide useful relief for minor irritations such as insect-bites. In a similar way, solutions of local anaesthetics may be infiltrated into a wound or applied to a mucous membrane, before minor surgery or dressing, and for the relief of continuing pain. Very commonly, a local anaesthetic (e.g. PRILOCAINE) is injected into a specific area, usually before beginning some procedure such as stitching a wound or dental operations, and here a VASOCONSTRICTOR agent, such as adrenaline, is often included to prolong the duration of action of the local anaesthesia by slowing the rate at which it is washed away by the bloodstream. The partial paralysis of movements of the lips and tongue that tends to accompany local anaesthesia in dentistry illustrates the fact that not only the nerves mediating sensation are affected, although fortunately, in practice, they are the first and most affected of the various nerve types.

For more invasive procedures, it may be necessary to paralyse all nerve fibres running from a region, perhaps a limb, and for this purpose the local anaesthetic is injected near a nerve trunk (*nerve block*). For producing a loss of sensation in a whole area of the body (for instance in childbirth, and for a wide variety of operations as an alternative to general anaesthesia when this is contra-indicated) the local anaesthetic may be injected into one of the spaces surrounding the spinal cord (*epidural*, *subdural* and *intrathecal* types of *spinal anaesthesia*). This type of procedure is carried out in the operating theatre, and the local anaesthetic (e.g. BUPIVACAINE) may be used as a 'heavy' preparation where the level of block in the spinal cord can be controlled by tilting the patient. The use of this procedure has been detailed above in relation to the control of pain in childbirth.

General anaesthetics

It is not appropriate to give much detail regarding the use of general anaesthetics, since it is both highly technical, with a number of drugs usually being used in concert, and also it is an area of which the patient is usually unaware and is rarely involved in choice. However, it may be noted that these agents are generally given either by intravenous injection or infusion, or inhalation. The former route may be used for induction purposes (e.g. with THIOPENTONE SODIUM) prior to inhalation anaesthesia, which normally allows greater control of effective dose. There are a number of volatile or gaseous anaesthetics, of which HALOTHANE is a common example. As already discussed, nitrous oxide, though having good analgesic properties, does not allow deep anaesthesia. Contrary to popular belief, ETHER is now rarely used in this country, and the use of chloroform was discontinued some time ago. General anaesthesia is now a much safer procedure than it used to be, one reason being that anaesthetists are now able to use a powerful array of drugs to achieve muscular relaxation (e.g. by nerve-muscle blocking agents such as d-tubocurarine, to control pain (e.g. with narcotic ANALGESICS), to produce sedation (e.g. with BENZODIAZEPINES or HYOSCINE, and to dry up secretions in the airways (e.g. with ANTICHOLINERGICS). The end result is that the patient does not need to be as deeply unconscious as of old, and indeed may even be aware of conversations in the operating theatre.

DRUGS USED IN TREATING SUBSTANCE DEPENDENCE

This is a specialized area, and can not be dealt with in any detail here though some remarks on addiction (*dependence*) to drugs is appropriate. It may be noted that continued use of a chemical can quite frequently lead to the individual adapting to the presence of the chemical, so there may be *tolerance* (a requirement to increase the dose to achieve the same effect), and a *withdrawal syndrome* on cessation of dosing. From what has been said in relation to the drug classes discussed above, it will be clear that dependence by habituation can occur with the medical use of drugs (e.g. BENZODIAZEPINES, narcotic ANALGESICS), as well as from the social or illegal use of chemicals (e.g. NICOTINE, ALCOHOL, HEROIN).

There are different types of therapy that are suitable for different purposes. In the event of the wish to give up an established addiction/habituation, the most straightforward course of action is to gradually decrease dosage (so as to minimize the withdrawal syndrome, see MINOR TRANQUILLIZERS, above) or substitute a less habituating and more easily managed drug (e.g. METHADONE for DIAMORPHINE – heroin). Once the individual has successfully withdrawn there may still be a danger of remission. Then it may be appropriate to give a drug that makes the subject feel unwell if the habituating substance is taken (e.g. DISULFIRAM for alcohol habituation). Lastly, receptor antagonists can be used either to treat an acute and life-threatening overdose (e.g. NALOXONE for opiate overdose) or to nullify the effects of a chemical and so discourage the taking of the habituating drug (e.g. NALTREXONE for opiate habituation).

In practice, stopping taking such drugs after becoming habituated is never easy, even when the subject seems quite resolute. In this respect, support groups and psychotherapeutic counselling can be very necessary.

PROSPECTS FOR THE FUTURE

Clearly, in this Introduction it has been possible only to touch on many areas worthy of chapters in their own right. The brain and its workings are undoubtedly among the most fascinating of all topics and the contribution of neuroscientists to our understanding of its mysteries is likely to become greater rather than less. In this endeavour, the investigation of the effects and actions of drugs on the brain has played, and will continue to play, an important role. As knowledge advances so do the prospects for successful treatment. To the author himself, it seems unlikely that psychoactive drugs will, in the foreseeable future, have the specificity and subtlety to be able to 'cure' conditions such as depression and schizophrenia; however, better control and less risk of side-effects seem eminently achievable. Another development to note is that the powerful techniques of molecular-genetics are raising the possibility that what seem bewilderingly complex disorders, such as manic-depressive illness and Alzheimer's disease, may be due to highly specific genetic lesions. Even in schizophrenia, that most destructive of psychiatric conditions, there have been inklings of links with physical abnormalities of brain structure or early infections. Such factors may be avoidable or treatable, providing the hope that future generations, by appropriate action, may greatly reduce their chances of developing such conditions. Inevitably there will be further false dawns, but such is the pace of neuroscience the promise of better treatments to come seems assured.

Dr John Halliday
Lecturer in Pharmacology
King's College London

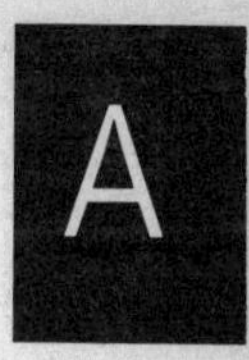

acetazolamide is a mildly diuretic (increases the flow of urine) drug used occasionally to treat some types of epilepsy including atypical absence seizures. Administration is oral in the form of tablets or capsules. Sodium and/or potassium supplements may be required during treatment.
▲ side-effects: there may be drowsiness, numbness and tingling of the hands and feet, flushes and headache, thirst, and frequency of urination.
⬢ warning: acetazolamide should not be administered to patients with sodium or potassium deficiency, or with malfunction of the adrenal glands, and should be administered with caution to patients who are pregnant or lactating, diabetic, or who have gout. Monitoring of the blood count and of electrolyte levels is essential.
Related article: DIAMOX.

Actifed Compound Linctus (*Wellcome*) is a proprietary, non-prescription, compound cough preparation, which is not available from the National Health Service. Produced in the form of an elixir for dilution (the elixir once dilute retains potency for 14 days), the Compound Linctus contains the sympathomimetic vasoconstrictor ephedrine, the sedative ANTIHISTAMINE triprolidine, and the NARCOTIC ANTITUSSIVE dextromethorphan.
▲/⬢ side-effects/warning: *see* DEXTROMETHORPHAN.

Acupan (*Carnegie*) is a proprietary, non-narcotic ANALGESIC, available only on prescription, used to treat moderate pain (such as that following minor surgery, or with toothache). Produced in the form of tablets and in ampoules for injection, Acupan is a preparation of nefopam hydrochloride.
▲/⬢ side-effects/warning: *see* NEFOPAM.

Adifax (*Servier*) is an APPETITE SUPPRESSANT, and is a proprietary form of dexfenfluramine hydrochloride, used to treat obesity, available only on prescription. The preparation is available in the form of capsules.
▲/⬢ side-effects/warning: *see* FENFLURAMINE HYDROCHLORIDE.
Related article: PONDERAX.

***adrenaline** is a HORMONE (a catecholamine) produced and secreted (along with smaller amounts of the closely related substance NORADRENALINE) by the central core (medulla) of the adrenal gland into the bloodstream. Together with noradrenaline these mediators are to a large part involved in orchestrating the body's response to activity and stress. Blood pressure is raised, the heart beats faster, and the metabolism is increased. Many of these SYMPATHOMIMETIC responses are associated with stress, especially palpitations and muscle tremor. These reactions may be treated with BETA-BLOCKERS.

Akineton (*Abbott*) is a proprietary preparation of the ANTI-CHOLINERGIC drug biperiden, available only on prescription, used to relieve some of the symptoms of parkinsonism (*see* ANTIPARKINSONIAN), specifically tremor of the hands, overall rigidity of posture, and the tendency to produce an excess of saliva. It is thought to work by compensating for the lack of dopamine in the brain, which is the major cause of such parkinsonian symptoms, and is produced in the form of tablets and in ampoules for injection.

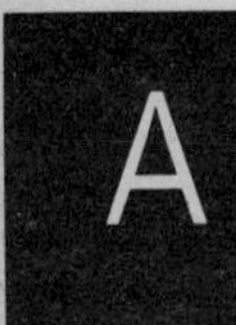

▲/✚ side-effects/warning: *see* BIPERIDEN.

alcohol is the name of a class of chemical compounds derived from hydrocarbons. Alcohol, in common usage, usually means ethyl alcohol (also called ethanol). For medical purposes, a strong solution of ethyl alcohol (surgical spirit) can be used both as an ANTISEPTIC (e.g. to prepare skin before injection) and as a preservative or solvent in many drug formulations.

As industrial alcohol it is commonly used as a general solvent, and both in this form and as Surgical Spirit it is 'denatured' by the addition of 5% methyl alcohol and substances with an unpleasant taste or smell to deter ingestion. However, methyl alcohol is highly toxic, so those who do drink such methylated spirits will suffer toxic reactions that include: palpitations, nausea, severe headache, and in higher doses loss of sight, bodily collapse, and even death.

Ethyl alcohol is the 'intoxicating' ingredient of fermented beverages such as beer and wine, which contain 5–15% alcohol, and distilled spirits, which contain about 50% ('100% proof' spirit is only about 50% ethyl alcohol). Ethyl alcohol (without contamination by methyl or other alcohols) is pharmacologically relatively safe when ingested in amounts up to the legal maximum blood concentration for driving (80 mg ethanol per 100 ml of blood). In amounts producing 2–4 times this blood concentration it has serious depressant actions on the brain centres, which are involved in the control of respiration and blood pressure. Very high dosages can result in coma and death. Other short-term effects include vomiting and flushing due to dilation of the blood vessels of the skin, this effect in a cold environment can lead to a dangerous (potentially fatal) loss of heat and hypothermia (fall in body temperature). Pharmacologically, alcohol is regarded as a depressant, and the apparent stimulant effect on behaviour may be regarded as a suppression of usual social inhibitions.

Long-term over-indulgence in alcoholic drinks can lead to serious and potentially fatal diseases including pancreatitis and cirrhosis of the liver. Ethyl alcohol is a habituating (addictive) drug, which leads to both tolerance (an increase in dose to achieve the same effect) and a withdrawal syndrome (adverse physical and psychological reaction on ceasing ingestion). In the treatment of alcoholism, if the subject successfully withdraws from alcohol and wishes for reinforcement in maintaining that state, then the drug DISULFIRAM (ANTABUSE) may be taken on a regular basis. This drug produces very unpleasant symptoms if any alcohol is ingested.

Other alcohols and related chemicals that are used as constituents of medical preparations include isopropyl alcohol, alcohol esters, and glycerol (glycerine).

alfentanil is a narcotic ANALGESIC of the OPIATE type, with a very short duration of action. It is used for short surgical operations, for outpatient surgery, or in combination to enhance the effect of general ANAESTHETIC (particularly barbiturate) drugs. Administration is by intravenous infusion, and may be continuous during prolonged surgical procedures. Its proprietary form is on the controlled drugs list.

▲ side-effects: there may be

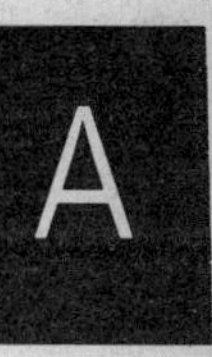

respiratory depression (severely shallow breathing), worsened by nausea and vomiting; the heart rate may slow and blood pressure fall.

● warning: respiration may become depressed during and following treatment; the use of alfentanil to assist with childbirth may lead to respiratory depression in the newborn. Alfentanil should therefore be administered with caution to patients who already suffer from respiratory disorders. Dosage should be reduced for the elderly and for patients who suffer from chronic liver disease.
Related article: RAPIFEN.

Alka-Donna-P (*Carlton*) is a form of the proprietary ANTI-CHOLINERGIC compound Alka-Donna, which is not available from the National Health Service, and is on the cotrolled drugs list because it additionally contains the BARBITURATE phenobarbitone.
▲/● side-effects/warning: *see* PHENOBARBITONE.

Allegron (*Dista*) is a proprietary TRICYCLIC ANTIDEPRESSANT, available only on prescription, used to treat depressive illness. It is also used for children to stop bed-wetting at night. Produced in the form of tablets (in two strengths), Allegron is a preparation of the drug nortriptyline hydrochloride.
▲/● side-effects/warning: *see* NORTRIPTYLINE.

Almazine (*Steinhard Cox*) is a proprietary ANXIOLYTIC, used as a tranquillizer especially in relieving attacks of phobia. Produced in the form of tablets (in two strengths), Almazine is a preparation of the relatively short-acting BENZODIAZEPINE lorazepam.
▲/● side-effects/warning: *see* LORAZEPAM.

aloxipirin is a non-narcotic ANALGESIC. It is a form of aspirin that additionally contains a buffer (a substance that counters acidity). This means that aspirin's detrimental effect on the lining of the stomach is somewhat reduced.
▲/● side-effects/warning: *see* ASPIRIN.
Related article: PALAPRIN FORTE.

alprazolam is an ANXIOLYTIC drug, one of the BENZODIAZEPINES used to treat anxiety in the short-term. Administration is oral in the form of tablets. It is not recommended for children.

▲ side-effects: there may be drowsiness, unsteadiness, headache, and shallow breathing; hypersensitivity reactions may occur.

● warning: alprazolam may reduce a patient's concentration and intricacy of movement or thought; it may also enhance the effects of alcohol consumption. Prolonged use or abrupt withdrawal should be avoided. It should be administered with caution to patients who suffer from respiratory difficulties, glaucoma, or kidney or liver disorders; who are in the last stages of pregnancy; or who are elderly or debilitated.
Related article: XANAX.

Alrheumat (*Bayer*) is a proprietary, non-steroid, ANTI-INFLAMMATORY, non-narcotic ANALGESIC drug, available only on prescription. It is used to relieve pain – particularly arthritic and rheumatic pain – and to treat other musculo-skeletal disorders. Its active constituent is ketoprofen, and it is produced in the form of capsules and anal suppositories.

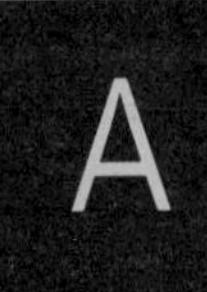

▲/✚ side-effects/warning: *see* KETOPROFEN.

amantadine hydrochloride is a drug used to treat parkinsonism (*see* ANTIPARKINSONIAN), but not the parkinsonian side-effects of other drugs. It is available on prescription only. Although not all patients respond to its use and tolerance develops, it has relatively few side-effects.

▲ side-effects: there may be insomnia, convulsions, nervousness, unsteadiness, hallucinations, skin discoloration, dry mouth, lack of concentration, swelling, and occasionally leucopenia (reduction in the number of white blood cells).

✚ warning: amantadine hydrochloride should not be administered to patients who have gastric ulceration, or who are epileptic. It should be given with caution to those with liver, kidney, or cardiovascular disease; who are elderly, lactating, or psychotic; or who suffer from recurrent eczema. Driving ability may also be impaired.

Related articles: MANTADINE; SYMMETREL.

amethocaine hydrochloride is a local ANAESTHETIC used in creams and in solution for topical application or instillation into the bladder, and in eye-drops for ophthalmic treatment. It is absorbed rapidly from mucous membrane surfaces.

▲ side-effects: rarely, there are hypersensitivity reactions.

✚ warning: topical administration may cause initial stinging. It should be given with caution to patients with epilepsy, impaired cardiac conduction or respiratory damage, or with liver damage.

Related article: NOXYFLEX.

amitriptyline is a TRICYCLIC ANTIDEPRESSANT drug that also has sedative properties. The sedation may be a benefit to agitated or violent patients, or to those who care for them. In contrast to the treatment of depressive illness, however, the drug may be used to prevent bed-wetting at night in youngsters. Administration is oral in the form of tablets, capsules or a dilute mixture. It is not recommended for young children.

▲ side-effects: common effects include sedation (affecting driving ability), dry mouth and blurred vision; there may also be difficulty in urinating, sweating and irregular heartbeat, behavioural disturbances, a rash, a state of confusion, and/or a loss of libido. Rarely, there are also blood disorders.

✚ warning: amitriptyline should not be administered to patients who suffer from heart disease or psychosis; it should be administered with caution to patients who suffer from diabetes, epilepsy, liver or thyroid disease, glaucoma or urinary retention; or who are pregnant or lactating. Withdrawal of treatment must be gradual.

Related articles: DOMICAL; ELAVIL; LENTIZOL; TRYPTIZOL.

amoxapine is a TRICYCLIC ANTIDEPRESSANT drug used to treat depressive illness.

▲ side-effects: common effects include sedation (affecting driving ability), dry mouth and blurred vision; there may also be difficulty in urinating, sweating and irregular heartbeat, behavioural disturbances, rashes, a state of confusion, menstrual irregularities, breast enlargement, and change in

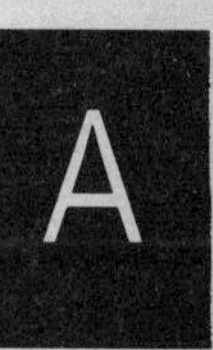

libido. Rarely, there are also blood disorders.
- warning: amoxapine should not be administered to patients who suffer from heart disease or psychosis; it should be administered with caution to patients who suffer from diabetes, epilepsy, liver or thyroid disease, glaucoma or urinary retention; or who are pregnant or lactating. Withdrawal of treatment must be gradual.
Related article: ASENDIS.

amylobarbitone is a BARBITURATE, used only when absolutely necessary as a HYPNOTIC to treat severe and intractable insomnia. Administration is oral in the form of tablets and capsules, or (as amylobarbitone sodium) by injection. Proprietary forms are all on the controlled drugs list.
- ▲ side-effects: concentration and the speed of movement and thought are affected. There may be drowsiness, dizziness and shallow breathing, with headache. Some patients experience hypersensitivity reactions. The drug may enhance the effects of alcohol consumption.
- warning: amylobarbitone should not be administered to patients whose insomnia is caused by pain, who have porphyria, who are pregnant or lactating, who are elderly or debilitated, or who have a history of drug (including alcohol) abuse. It should be administered with caution to those with kidney, liver or lung disease. Use of the drug should be avoided as far as possible. Repeated doses are cumulative in effect, and may lead to real sedation; abrupt withdrawal of treatment, on the other hand, may cause serious withdrawal symptoms. Tolerance and dependence (addiction) occur readily.
Related articles: AMYTAL; SECONAL SODIUM; SODIUM AMYTAL; TUINAL.

Amytal (*Lilly*) is a proprietary HYPNOTIC drug, a BARBITURATE, and on the controlled drugs list; it is used to treat persistent and intractable insomnia. A dangerous and potentially addictive drug, it is produced in the form of tablets (in five strengths) and is a preparation of amylobarbitone. It is not recommended for children.
- ▲/ side-effects/warning: *see* AMYLOBARBITONE.

Anadin (*Whitehall Laboratories*) is a proprietary, non-prescription compound, non-narcotic ANALGESIC produced in the form of tablets and as capsules. Anadin is a preparation of aspirin, caffeine and quinine sulphate.
- ▲/ side-effects/warning: *see* ASPIRIN; CAFFEINE.

Anadin Extra (*Whitehall Laboratories*) is a proprietary, non-prescription compound, non-narcotic ANALGESIC produced in the form of tablets and as capsules. Anadin is a preparation of aspirin, caffeine and paracetamol.
- ▲/ side-effects/warning: *see* ASPIRIN; CAFFEINE; PARACETOMOL.

***anaesthetic** is a drug that reduces sensation; such drugs affect either a specific local area – a local anaesthetic – or the whole body with loss of consciousness – a general anaesthetic. A drug used to induce general anaesthesia (i.e. bring about a smooth and rapid transition to the state of unconsciousness) is generally different from the drug or drugs used to maintain that state. Drugs used frequently to

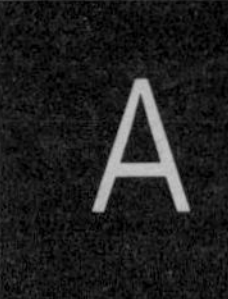

cause anaesthesia include THIOPENTONE SODIUM and ETOMIDATE. Used on their own these drugs are too short-acting to provide a useful period of surgical anaesthesia. Common drugs such as oxygen-nitrous oxide mixtures and HALOTHANE are used to maintain anaesthesia.

Before induction, a premedication is usually administered to a patient an hour or so before an operation. These premedications can have multiple pharmacological actions. They may contain a drug to calm the nerves, or to diminish salivary, tracheal and bronchial secretions, which might otherwise block respiratory passages. They often contain a long-acting analgesic, which covers the period during and after recovery from anaesthesia. Examples of such premedications include, ANTICHOLINERGICS, OPIATES and BENZODIAZEPINES.

During surgery other types of drug may be used in addition to general anaesthetics. For most internal surgery and whenever artificial respiration is employed a SKELETAL MUSCLE RELAXANT is also required.

Local anaesthetics are injected or absorbed in the area of the body where they are intended to take effect. They work by impairing temporarily the function of nerves serving or passing through the site. Frequently used local anaesthetics include LIGNOCAINE, which is widely used in dental surgery. One form of local anaesthesia, known as epidural anaesthesia, is produced by the injection of anaesthetic into the membranes surrounding the spinal cord, which causes numbness from the abdomen down. 'Epidurals' are often used to control pain during labour. Local anaesthetics commonly used to produce epidural anaesthetic are LIGNOCAINE and BUPIVACAINE HYDROCHLORIDE.

Anafranil (*Geigy*) is a proprietary ANTIDEPRESSANT, available only on prescription, used to relieve the symptoms of depressive illness and as an additional treatment in phobic and obsessional states. It is also used to treat attacks of muscular weakness that occur in narcolepsy. Produced in the form of capsules (in three strengths), as sustained-release tablets (under the name Anafranil SR), as a syrup (the potency of the dilute syrup lasts for 7 days), and in ampoules for injection, Anafranil is a preparation of the tricyclic antidepressant clomipramine hydrochloride. None of these preparations is recommended for children.

▲/♣ side-effects/warning: *see* CLOMIPRAMINE HYDROCHLORIDE.

***analgesic** is a drug that relieves pain. Because pain is a subjective experience that can arise from many causes, there are many ways that drugs can be used to relieve it. However, the term analgesic is best restricted to two main classes of drug.

First, NARCOTIC analgesics are drugs such as MORPHINE, which have powerful actions on the central nervous system and alter the transmission and perception of pain. Because of the numerous possible side-effects, perhaps the most well-known is drug dependence (addiction), this class is usually used under medical supervision, and normally the drugs are only available on prescription. Other notable side-effects commonly include depression of respiration, nausea and sometimes hypotension, constipation, inhibition of coughing, and constriction of the pupils. Other notable members of this class include DIAMORPHINE

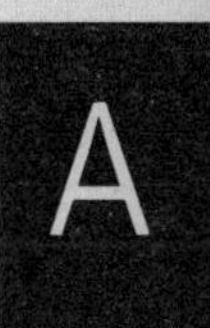

(heroin), PENTAZOCINE, METHADONE, PETHIDINE and CODEINE, in descending order of their potency to deal with severe pain.

Second, non-narcotic analgesics are drugs such as ASPIRIN, which have no tendency to produce dependence, but are by no means free of side-effects. This class is referred to by many names, including weak analgesics and, in medical circles, NSAIDs (non-steroidal anti-inflammatory drugs). The latter term refers to the valuable ANTI-INFLAMMATORY action of some members of the class (a property shared with the corticosteroids). This class of drug is used for a variety of purposes, ranging from mild aches and pains (at normal dosage) to the treatment of rheumatoid arthritis (at higher dosage). PARACETAMOL does not have strong anti-inflammatory actions, but, as with other drugs in this class, has the valuable ability to lower raised body temperature (ANTIPYRETIC action). In spite of these important actions and uses, all members of the class have side-effects of concern, which for aspirin-like drugs include gastrointestinal upsets ranging from dyspepsia to serious haemorrhage. Other examples of drugs of this class include IBUPROFEN and INDOMETHACIN. Often drugs in this class are used in combination with each other (e.g. paracetamol and codeine) or with drugs of other classes (e.g. caffeine).

Apart from these two main classes, there are other drugs that are sometimes referred to as analgesics because of their ability to relieve pain (e.g. local anaesthetics are known as local analgesics in the USA). To achieve the degree of pain relief necessary for major surgical operations general ANAESTHETICS are used, but often in conjunction with narcotic analgesics.

Anethaine (*Evans*) is a proprietary, non-prescription local ANAESTHETIC, used to treat painful skin conditions and itching. Produced in the form of a water-miscible cream for topical application, Anethaine is a preparation of amethocaine hydrochloride.
▲/ ● side-effects/warning: *see* AMETHOCAINE.

Anexate (*Roche*) is a BENZODIAZEPINE antagonist used to reverse the central sedative effects of benzodiazepines in anaesthesia, intensive care and diagnostic procedures. Administration is by injection or slow intravenous infusion.
▲/ ● side-effects/warning: *see* FLUMAZENIL.

Angettes 75 (*Bristol-Myers*) is a proprietary, low-dose preparation of the ANTI-INFLAMMATORY, non-narcotic ANALGESIC drug aspirin, used here to reduce blood platelet adhesion, and thus formation of blood clots (thrombi). It is particularly indicated after problems relating to blocked blood vessels, such as myocardial infarction. Angettes is available without prescription, in the form of tablets.
▲/ ● side-effects/warning: *see* ASPIRIN.

Anquil (*Janssen*) is a proprietary ANTIPSYCHOTIC drug, available only on prescription, used to treat psychosis (especially schizophrenia) and as a major TRANQUILLIZER in patients undergoing behavioural disturbance. It is used to treat deviant and antisocial sexual behaviour. Produced in the form of tablets, Anquil is a preparation of the butyrophenone drug

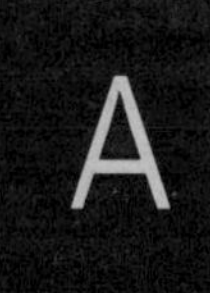

benperidol. It is not recommended for children.
▲/♣ side-effects/warning: *see* BENPERIDOL.

Antabuse (*CP Pharmaceuticals*) is a proprietary preparation of the drug disulfiram, available only on prescription. It is used as an adjunct in the treatment of alcoholism because, in combination with the consumption of even small quantities of alcohol, it gives rise to unpleasant reactions – such as flushing, headache, palpitations, nausea and vomiting. Produced in the form of tablets, Antabuse is not recommended for children.
▲/♣ side-effects/warning: *see* DISULFIRAM.

***anticholinergic** drugs inhibit the action, release or production of the substance acetylcholine (a NEUROTRANSMITTER), which plays an important role in the nervous system. Such drugs tend to relax smooth muscle, reduce the secretion of saliva, digestive juices and sweat, and to dilate the pupil of the eye. They may thus be used as antispasmodics, or in the treatment of parkinsonian symptoms or of peptic ulcers, and in ophthalmic examinations. However, use of such drugs is commonly accompanied by side-effects, including dry mouth, dry skin, blurred vision, an increased heart rate, constipation and difficulty in urinating. Examples of anticholinergic drugs include ATROPINE, HYOSCINE and BENZHEXOL HYDROCHLORIDE.

***anticonvulsant** drugs prevent the onset of epileptic seizures or reduce their severity if they do occur. Among the most widely used is SODIUM VALPROATE, which is used to treat all common forms of epilepsy. Other anticonvulsants include those used solely to treat grand mal forms of epilepsy (e.g. CARBAMAZEPINE and PHENYTOIN), and those used to treat petit mal forms of epilepsy (e.g. ETHOSUXIMIDE). In every case dosage must be adjusted to the requirements of the patient.

***antidepressants** are drugs that relieve the symptoms of depressive illness. There are three main groups of drugs used for the purpose. One is the group nominally called tricyclic antidepressants, which include AMITRIPTYLINE, IMIPRAMINE and DOXEPIN, and these are effective in alleviating a number of the symptoms – although they have anticholinergic side-effects. Tricyclic antidepressants are often useful in the treatment of a specific anxiety state called panic disorder.

The second 'group' consists of the monoamine-oxidase inhibitors (MAOIs), including for example ISOCARBOXAZID, TRANYLCYPROMINE and PHENELZINE. These are now used less frequently because they have severe side-effects.

The 'third' group is a miscellany of drugs all possessing some antidepressant activity, but seemingly of different mechanisms of action. Mianserin, trazodone and fluoxetine might be considered in this category. Caution must be taken in prescribing antidepressant drugs.

***anti-emetic**, or antinauseant, drugs prevent vomiting, and are therefore used primarily to prevent travel sickness, to relieve vertigo experienced by patients with infection of the organs of balance in the ears, or to alleviate nausea in patients undergoing irradiation therapy or chemotherapy for cancer. The range of drugs that possess some anti-emetic activity is large. Most of the ANTIHISTAMINES, for instance, are mildly effective.

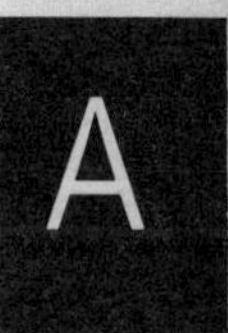

HYOSCINE is also useful, and in many cases so are the PHENOTHIAZINE derivatives such as CHLORPROMAZINE and PROCHLORPERAZINE. More recently METOCLOPRAMIDE, DOMPERIDONE and ONDANSETRON have been found to be very useful in treating severe emesis brought on by cytotoxic drugs. In all cases treatment causes drowsiness and reduces concentration, and enhances the effects of alcohol consumption. Anti-emetic drugs should not be administered to treat vomiting in pregnancy, and most are not cleared for this use.

***anti-epileptic** drugs are more usually described as anticonvulsant drugs (even though some forms of epilepsy may not cause convulsions). *see* ANTICONVULSANT.

***antihistamines** are drugs that inhibit the effects in the body of histamine. Such a release occurs naturally as the result of a patient's coming into contact with a substance to which he or she is allergic, and the resultant symptoms may be those of hay fever, urticaria, itching (pruritus) or bronchoconstriction. Many antihistamines also have sedative and ANTI-EMETIC properties, and may be used to prevent travel sickness, vertigo, or (less effectively) nausea and vomiting caused by chemotherapy in the treatment of cancer. Side-effects following administration of antihistamines commonly include drowsiness, dizziness, blurred vision, gastrointestinal disturbances and a lack of muscular co-ordination.

Conventionally, only the earlier discovered drugs that act on histamine's H_1 receptors are referred to by the general name 'antihistamines'. Somewhat confusingly, however, the recently discovered drugs widely used in the treatment of peptic ulcers (e.g. cimetidine and ranitidine) are also antihistamines, but act on another class of receptor (H_2) that is involved in gastric secretion. The following list are examples of traditional H_1 antihistamines with sedative or anti-emetic actions:
CINNARIZINE; CYCLIZINE; DIMENHYDRINATE; DIPHENHYDRAMINE HYDROCHLORIDE; PROMETHAZINE HYDROCHLORIDE.

***anti-inflammatory** drugs are those used to reduce inflammation (the body's defensive reaction when tissue is injured). The way they work depends on the type of drug (e.g. corticosteroid or NSAID), but may involve actions such as the reduction of blood flow or white blood cell response in the inflamed area, or an inhibitory effect on the chemicals released in the tissue that cause the inflammation.

***antimigraine** drugs are used to treat the frequency of occurance or the unpleasant effects of migraine attacks. A number of different types of drug are used, including ERGOTAMINE, PIZOTIFEN and a number of ANALGESIC preparations.

***antinauseants** are usually described as anti-emetics, since in practice most drugs that remedy nausea (the sensation that makes people feel as if they are about to vomit) also prevent vomiting. *see* ANTI-EMETIC.

***antiparkinsonian** drugs are used to treat parkinsonism, the primary cause of which is the central neurodegenerative condition called Parkinson's Disease. This produces symptoms of poverty and difficulty in

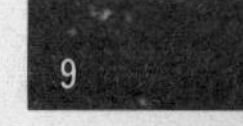

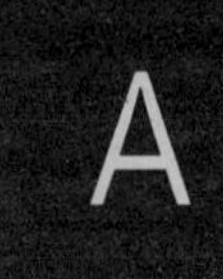

initiating movement, muscle tremor and rigidity (extra-pyramidal symptoms), especially in the limbs. It results from a deficiency of the neurotransmitter DOPAMINE in a particular nerve pathway in the brain (the nigro-striatal tract). This appears to produce an imbalance of the actions of DOPAMINE and other neurotransmitters (e.g. acetylcholine) in important extrapyramidal centres controlling movement in the brain. Most interestingly, parkinsonian extrapyramidal side-effects may be caused by treatment with several types of drugs, especially the ANTI-PSYCHOTICS (e.g. HALOPERIDOL). Treatment of parkinsonism used to be restricted to ANTICHOLINERGIC drugs (e.g. BENZHEXOL), but now drugs that increase the synthesis of dopamine (e.g. LEVODOPA), or replace it (e.g. BROMOCRIPTINE), or otherwise enhance its activity (e.g. AMANTIDINE) are used to greater effect. The former class, anticholinergics, are more useful for controlling fine tremor (including that induced by drugs) and the latter class for over-coming difficulty in commencing movement. Overcompensation with some of the replacement therapies may be a problem and a good balance of effect can be difficult to achieve.

***antipsychotic** drugs, also known as NEUROLEPTICS or major TRANQUILLIZERS, are used to calm and sedate psychotic patients without impairing consciousness and, more importantly, to restore their thought processes to a more ordered state. The term psychosis refers to a severe mental disturbance associated with hallucinations, delusions and grossly distorted thought processes. These are characteristic features of the heterogeneous group of disorders commonly called schizophrenia.

Antipsychotics exert their effect by an action on the brain, it is thought primarily by depressing the activity of a neurotransmitter called DOPAMINE. Because this transmitter is invloved in many functions in the brain (and because the drugs also effect other neurotransmitter systems) antipsychotic agents can exhibit many side-effects, including, in the short-term, hormonal effects and movement disorders similar to those of Parkinson's disease. With chronic use they can cause a condition called 'tardive dyskinesias', which includes compulsive abnormal facial and oral movements, and restlessness.

Antipsychotic drugs include HALOPERIDOL, FLUPENTHIXOL DECANOATE and the PHENOTHIAZINE derivatives, particularly CHLORPROMAZINE and THIORIDAZINE. SULPIRIDE requires careful adjustment of dosage depending on effect, and BENPERIDOL is used mostly to control antisocial behaviour or hyperactivity.

***antipyretic** drugs reduce high body temperature. Best-known and most-used antipyretic drugs include the ANALGESICS ASPIRIN, PARACETAMOL and MEFENAMIC ACID.

***antitussives** are drugs that assist in the treatment of coughs. Generally the term antitussive is used to describe only those drugs that suppress coughing rather than drugs used to treat the cause of coughing. Cough suppressants include OPIATES such as DEXTROMETHORPHAN, PHOLCODINE and CODEINE. They tend to cause constipation as a side-effect and so should not be used for prolonged periods.

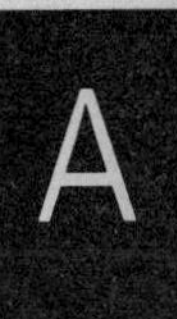

Antoin (*Cox*) is a proprietary, non-prescription compound ANALGESIC, which is not available from the National Health Service. Used to relieve mild to moderate pain anywhere in the body, and produced in the form of soluble (dispersible) tablets, Antoin is a preparation of aspirin with the OPIATE codeine phosphate and the mild STIMULANT caffeine citrate. It is not recommended for children.
▲/● side-effects/warning: *see* ASPIRIN; CAFFEINE; CODEINE PHOSPHATE.

***anxiolytic** drugs relieve anxiety states and should only be prescribed for patients whose anxiety in the face of stress (actual or perceived) is actually hindering the prospect of its resolution. Treatment should be at the lowest dosage effective, and must not be prolonged: psychological dependence (if not physical addiction) readily occurs and may make withdrawal difficult. Best-known and most widely prescribed anxiolytic drugs are the BENZODIAZEPINES, such as DIAZEPAM, CHLORDIAZEPOXIDE, LORAZEPAM and CLOBAZAM. The benzodiazepines are also frequently used as HYPNOTICS and are sometimes used in the relief of withdrawal symptoms caused by addiction to other drugs (such as alcohol). Drugs of this class may also be referred to as minor TRANQUILLIZERS. For cases where the anxiety has a prominent somatic (i.e. sensation of palpitations, sweating and tremor) rather than psychic component, beta adrenoceptor blockers such as propranolol have sometimes proved useful (e.g. public performance anxiety experienced by snooker players and musicians). In the specific anxiety states termed panic disorders tricyclic antidepressants may have a beneficial effect.

Apisate (*Wyeth*) is a proprietary APPETITE SUPPRESSANT, which is on the controlled drugs list. Produced in the form of sustained-release tablets, Apisate is a preparation of the amphetamine-related drug diethylpropion hydrochloride together with a vitamin supplement of thiamine (vitamin B_1), riboflavine (vitamin B_2), pyridoxine (vitamin B_6), and the B vitamin derivative nicotinamide. Treatment must be in the short-term and under strict medical supervision; the drug is not recommended for children.
▲/● side-effects/warning: *see* DIETHYLPROPION HYDROCHLORIDE.

***appetite suppressants** are intended to assist in the medical treatment of obesity – in which the primary therapy has to be in the form of diet. They work either by acting on the brain to depress the urge to eat or by bulking out the food eaten so that the body feels it has actually taken more than it has. Appetite suppressants that act on the brain include FENFLURAMINE HYDROCHLORIDE, DIETHYLPROPION HYDROCHLORIDE and PHENTERMINE. The latter two are amphetamine-like and are not recommended due to side-effects and problems of dependence and abuse.

Apsifen (*Approved Prescription Services*) is a proprietary, non-narcotic ANALGESIC, available only on prescription, used to relieve pain, particularly the pain of rheumatic disease and other musculo-skeletal disorders. It is produced in the form of tablets, which can be film- or sugar-coated; the film-coated are available in three strengths and the sugar-coated in two strengths.

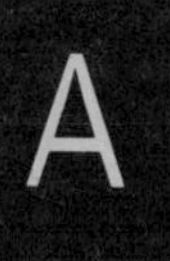

Apsifen is a preparation of the ANTI-INFLAMMATORY drug ibuprofen.
▲/✚ side-effects/warning: *see* IBUPROFEN.

Arpicolin (*RP Drugs*) is a proprietary preparation of the ANTICHOLINERGIC drug procyclidine hydrochloride, available only on prescription, used in the treatment of parkinsonism and to control tremors induced by drugs (*see* ANTIPARKINSONIAN). Produced in the form of a syrup (in two strengths), Arpicolin is not recommended for children.
▲/✚ side-effects/warning: *see* PROCYCLIDINE.

Artane (*Lederle*) is a proprietary preparation of the ANTICHOLINERGIC drug benzhexol hydrochloride, available only on prescription, used in the treatment of parkinsonism and to control tremors and involuntary movement. Produced in the form of tablets (in two strengths), and as a powder (for oral use). Artane is not recommended for children.
▲/✚ side-effects/warning: *see* BENZHEXOL HYDROCHLORIDE.

Arthroxen (*Cox, CP Pharmaceuticals Ltd*) is a proprietary form of the non-steroidal, ANTI-INFLAMMATORY (NSAID), non-narcotic ANALGESIC drug naproxen. Available on prescription only, it is used to treat pain and inflammation associated with rheumatic disease and other musculo-skeletal disorders. Administered in the form of tablets (in two strengths).
▲/✚ side-effects/warning: *see* NAPROXEN.

Artracin (*DDSA Pharmaceuticals*) is a non-proprietary, non-steroidal, ANTI-INFLAMMATORY non-narcotic ANALGESIC, available only on prescription, used to treat the pain of rheumatic and other musculo-skeletal disorders (including gout). Produced in the form of capsules (in two strengths), Artracin is a preparation of indomethacin. It is not recommended for children.
▲/✚ side-effects/warning: *see* INDOMETHACIN.

Asendis (*Lederle*) is a proprietary form of the TRICYCLIC ANTI-DEPRESSANT drug amoxapine, used to treat depressive illness. Available, only on prescription, in the form of tablets in three strengths.
▲/✚ side-effects/warning: *see* AMOXAPINE.

Aspav (*Cox*) is a proprietary compound ANALGESIC, available only on prescription, used to relieve pain, especially pain following surgery or caused by inoperable cancer. Produced in the form of dissolvable tablets, Aspav is a combination of aspirin and the OPIATE papaveretum. It is not recommended for children.
▲/✚ side-effects/warning: *see* ASPIRIN; PAPAVERETUM.

aspirin, or acetylsalicylic acid, is a well-known and widely used non-narcotic ANALGESIC, which has non-steroidal, ANTI-INFLAMMATORY properties and is useful in reducing high body temperature (ANTIPYRETIC). As an analgesic it relieves mild to moderate pain, particularly headache, toothache, menstrual pain and the aches of rheumatic disease. Its temperature-reducing capacity helps in the treatment of the common cold, fevers or influenza. Aspirin is also used as an ANTICOAGULANT. In tablet form, aspirin may irritate the stomach lining and many forms of soluble aspirin, in trying to avoid this drawback, include chalk. Other proprietary forms combine

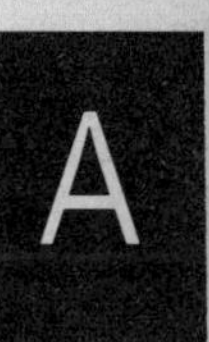

aspirin with such drugs as codeine or paracetamol. Administration is oral or, rarely, by injection. It is advised that aspirin should not be administered to children aged under 12 years, unless specially indicated. Some people are allergic to aspirin.

▲ side-effects: gastric irritation with or without haemorrhage is common, although such effects may be neutralized to some extent by taking the drug after food. Aspirin may enhance the effect of some hypoglycaemic and anticoagulant drugs.

⯃ warning: irritation of the stomach lining may, in susceptible patients, cause nausea, vomiting, pain and bleeding (which may lead to anaemia if prolonged). Overdosage may cause ringing in the ears (tinnitus), dizziness, nausea, vomiting, headache, hyperventilation, and sometimes a state of confusion or delirium followed by coma. Aspirin may also dispose a patient to bronchospasm, which in asthmatic patients may prove problematic. Repeated overdosage may result in kidney damage. *Related articles:* ANGETTES 75; ANTOIN; ASPAV; CAPRIN; CODIS; EQUAGESIC; HYPON; LABOPRIN; MIGRAVESS; NU-SEALS ASPIRIN; PALAPRIN FORTE; PLATET; ROBAXISAL FORTE; SOLPRIN; VEGANIN.

Atarax (*Pfizer*) is a proprietary ANTIHISTAMINE, available only on prescription. It is used to treat emotional disturbances and anxiety (*see* ANXIOLYTIC), which may manifest as physical symptoms. Atarax may be used as a SEDATIVE (e.g. before or after surgery), and as an ANTI-EMETIC. Produced in the form of tablets (in two strengths) and as a syrup (under the trade name Atarax Syrup), Atarax is a preparation of hydroxyzine hydrochloride.

▲/⯃ side-effects/warning: *see* HYDROXYZINE HYDROCHLORIDE.

Atensine (*Berk*) is a proprietary ANXIOLYTIC, available on prescription only to private patients, used both as an anxiolytic or minor TRANQUILLIZER (to treat states of anxiety, insomnia and nervous tension) and to relieve muscle spasm and cerebral palsy. It may also be used as a premedication for dental operations. Produced in the form of tablets (in three strengths), Atensine is a preparation of the BENZODIAZEPINE diazepam.

▲/⯃ side-effects/warning: *see* DIAZEPAM.

Ativan (*Wyeth*) is a proprietary ANXIOLYTIC, available only on prescription, used as an anxiolytic or minor TRANQUILLIZER (to treat anxiety, phobias, and as a HYPNOTIC in insomnia), and as a SEDATIVE or premedication before surgery. Produced in the form of tablets (in two strengths) and in ampoules for injection, Ativan represents a preparation of the relatively short-acting BENZODIAZEPINE lorazepam.

▲/⯃ side-effects/warning: *see* LORAZEPAM.

atropine is a powerful ANTICHOLINERGIC drug obtained from plants including belladonna (deadly nightshade). In combination with morphine it may be used as a premedication to inhibit salivary and bronchial secretions, and the motility of visceral organs during surgery. Administration is by injection.

▲ side-effects: there is commonly dry mouth and thirst; there may also be visual disturbances, and constipation.

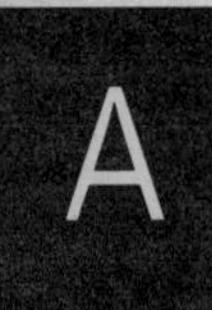

● warning: atropine should not be administered to patients with enlargement of the prostate gland.

Audax (*Napp*) is a proprietary, non-prescription, non-narcotic ANALGESIC in the form of ear-drops, used to soothe pain associated with infection of the outer or middle ear. Its active constituent is choline salicylate.

● warning: *see* CHOLINE SALICYLATE.

Aventyl (*Lilly*) is a proprietary tricyclic ANTIDEPRESSANT drug, available only on prescription, used to treat depressive illness – but also used to treat nocturnal bedwetting in children (although not recommended for children aged under 6 years or for treatment periods of longer than three months). Produced in the form of capsules (in two strengths), Aventyl represents a preparation of nortriptyline hydrochloride.

▲/● side-effects/warning: *see* NORTRIPTYLINE.

Avomine (*May & Baker*) is a proprietary, non-prescription ANTINAUSEANT drug used to treat symptoms of nausea, vomiting and/or vertigo caused by certain diseases, or motion sickness. Produced in the form of tablets, Avomine is a preparation of promethazine theoclate.

▲/● side-effects/warning: *see* PROMETHAZINE THEOCLATE.

azapropazone is a non-steroidal ANTI-INFLAMMATORY non-narcotic ANALGESIC, used primarily to treat rheumatic and arthritic complaints, gout, and musculo-skeletal pain. Administration is oral in the form of capsules and tablets. It is not recommended for children.

▲ side-effects: there is commonly a rash; there may also be a sensitivity to light. Sometimes there is accumulation of fluid within the tissues (oedema) and consequent weight gain. There may be gastrointestinal upsets.

● warning: azapropazone should not be administered to patients with peptic ulcer or impairment of kidney function, or who are taking sulphonamides; it should be administered with caution to those with impaired liver function or with allergic disorders, who are elderly, or who are pregnant. It should not be given to patients who are taking phenytoin, drugs that lower the blood sugar level, or anticoagulants.

baclofen is a drug, used as a SKELETAL MUSCLE RELAXANT, that relaxes muscles which are in spasm, especially muscles in the limbs, and particularly when caused by injury or disease in the central nervous system. Although it is chemically unrelated to any other ANTISPASMODIC drug, it has similar clinical uses to certain of the benzodiazepine group of drugs. It acts by activating a specific set of inhibtory neurotransmitter receptors in the spinal cord. Administration is oral in the form of tablets or a dilute sugar-free liquid.

▲ side-effects: there may be drowsiness and fatigue, weakness and low blood pressure (hypotension); elderly or debilitated patients may enter a state of confusion. Nausea and vomiting may occur.

● warning: baclofen should be administered with caution to patients with impaired cerebrovascular system, epilepsy, or psychiatric conditions, or who are elderly. Initial dosage should be gradually increased (to avoid sedation); withdrawal of treatment should be equally gradual.

barbiturates are a group of drugs derived from barbituric acid, with a wide range of essentially depressent actions. They are now used mostly as general ANAESTHETICS. They work by direct action on the brain, depressing specific centres, and may be slow- or fast-acting; all are extremely effective. However, all also quite rapidly produce tolerance and then both psychological and physical dependence, and for that reason are used as sparingly as possible for any extended use. An accidental or intentional overdose of barbiturate tablets can be fatal. Best-known and most-used barbiturates include the anticonvulsant phenobarbitone, and the very short-acting general anaesthetics thiopentone and methohexitone. Administration is oral in the form of tablets, or by intravenous injection.

▲ side-effects: there is drowsiness and dizziness with a hangover effect; there may be shallow breathing and headache. Some patients experience sensitivity reactions that may be serious.

● warning: barbiturates should be avoided wherever possible. They should not in any case be administered to patients who suffer from insomnia caused by pain or from porphyria, who are pregnant or lactating, who are elderly, debilitated or very young, or who have a history of drug or alcohol abuse (barbiturates greatly enhance the effects of alcohol). Barbiturates should be administered with caution to those with kidney or liver disease, or impaired lung function. Prolonged use should be avoided, as should abrupt withdrawal of treatment (which might lead to withdrawal symptoms). Tolerance develops when barbiturates are taken repeatedly, an increasingly larger dose being necessary to produce the same effect; continued use leads to psychological and physical dependence.
see AMYLOBARBITONE; BUTOBARBITONE; METHOHEXITONE SODIUM; METHYLPHENOBARBITONE; PHENOBARBITONE; QUINALBARBITONE SODIUM; THIOPENTONE SODIUM.

Beecham's Powders (*Beecham Health Care*) is a proprietary, non-

prescription cold relief preparation. It contains paracetamol, caffeine and ascorbic acid.
▲/ ⬢ side-effects/warning: *see* CAFFEINE; PARACETAMOL.

Benadryl (*Parke-Davis*) is a proprietary, non-prescription ANTIHISTAMINE. It has ANTINAUSEANT properties and is used to treat or prevent travel sickness, vertigo and infections of the inner or middle ear. Produced in the form of capsules, Benadryl is a preparation of the somewhat SEDATIVE antihistamine diphenhydramine hydrochloride. It is not recommended for children.
▲/ ⬢ side-effects/warning: *see* DIPHENHYDRAMINE HYDROCHLORIDE.

Benoral (*Sterling Research*) is a proprietary, non-prescription non-narcotic ANALGESIC used to treat mild to moderate pain, especially the pain of rheumatic disease and other musculo-skeletal disorders. Produced in the form of tablets, as a powder in sachets for solution, and as a sugar-free suspension for dilution (the potency of the suspension once dilute is retained for 14 days), Benoral is a preparation of an ester derived from both ASPIRIN and PARACETAMOL called benorylate.
▲/ ⬢ side-effects/warning: *see* BENORYLATE.

benorylate is a non-narcotic ANALGESIC, with both ANTI-INFLAMMATORY and ANTIPYRETIC actions, which breaks down chemically after gastrointestinal absorption to ASPIRIN and PARACETAMOL. It is used particularly to treat the pain of rheumatic disease and other musculo-skeletal disorders, and to lower a high temperature. Administration is oral in the form of tablets, a solution or a dilute suspension.
▲ side-effects: gastrointestinal disturbance is fairly common, but there may also be nausea and bleeding. Some patients experience hearing disturbances and vertigo. A few proceed to hyper-sensitivity reactions, blood disorders, or a state of confusion. Prolonged use or overdosage may cause liver damage.
⬢ warning: benorylate should not be administered to patients intolerant of aspirin, with peptic ulcers, who are already taking aspirin or paracetamol in some other form, or who are aged under 12 years. It should be administered with caution to those with allergic conditions, who have impaired kidney or liver function, who suffer from alcoholism, or from dehydration; who are elderly; who are pregnant or lactating; or who are already taking anticoagulant drugs.
Related article: BENORAL.

benperidol is a powerful ANTIPSYCHOTIC drug, used to treat and tranquillize psychotic patients, especially suitable for treating antisocial and deviant forms of sexual behaviour. Administration is oral in the form of tablets. It is not recommended for children.
▲ side-effects: sedation and extrapyramidal symptoms are likely to occur. Muscles in the neck and back, and sometimes the arms, may undergo spasms. There may also be restlessness, insomnia and nightmares; rashes and jaundice may appear; and there may be dry mouth, gastrointestinal disturbance, difficulties in urinating, and blurred vision. Long-term use may give rise to irreversible movement disorders (tardive dyskinesias). Rarely, there is weight loss and

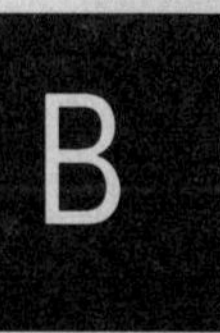

impaired kidney function.

✚ warning: benperidol should not be administered to patients who have a reduction in the bone-marrow's capacity to produce blood cells, or certain types of glaucoma. It should be administered only with caution to those with heart or vascular disease, kidney or liver disease, parkinsonism, or depression; or who are pregnant or lactating.
Related article: ANQUIL.

benserazide is an enzyme inhibitor that is administered therapeutically in combination with the drug levodopa to treat parkinsonism, but not the parkinsonian symptoms induced by drugs (*see* ANTIPARKINSONIAN). The benserazide prevents too rapid a breakdown in the body of the levodopa (into dopamine), allowing more levodopa to reach the brain to make up the deficiency (of dopamine) that is the major cause of parkinsonian symptoms. Administration of the combination is oral in the form of capsules.

▲/✚ side-effects/warning: complex mode of action makes side-effects and interactions with many other drugs likely, so great care should be taken in its use. Also *see* LEVODOPA.
Related article: MADOPAR.

Bentex (*Steinhard*) is a proprietary preparation of the drug benzhexol hydrochloride, available only on prescription, used to relieve some of the symptoms of parkinsonism (*see* ANTIPARKINSONIAN), specifically tremor, overall rigidity of posture, and the tendency to produce an excess of saliva. (The drug also has the capacity to treat these conditions in some cases where they are produced by drugs.) It is thought to work by compensating indirectly for the lack of dopamine in the brain that is the major cause of such parkinsonian symptoms. Bentex is produced in the form of tablets (in two strengths), to be taken before or after food. Counselling of patients is advised.

▲/✚ side-effects/warning: *see* BENZHEXOL HYDROCHLORIDE.

benzhexol hydrochloride is an ANTICHOLINERGIC agent employed in the treatment of some types of parkinsonism (*see* ANTIPARKINSONIAN). It decreases rigidity and has a limited effect on tremors. The tendency to produce an excess of saliva is also reduced by benzhexol. (The drug also has the capacity to treat these conditions in some cases where they are produced by drugs.) It is thought to work by compensating for the lack of dopamine in the brain, which is the major cause of such parkinsonian symptoms, by reducing the cholinergic excess. Administration – which may be in parallel with the administration of other drugs used for the relief of parkinsonism – is oral in the form of tablets or sustained-release capsules, or as a dilute syrup.

▲ side-effects: there may be dry mouth, dizziness and blurred vision, and/or gastrointestinal disturbances. Some patients experience sensitivity reactions and anxiety. Rarely, and in susceptible patients, there may be confusion, agitation and psychological disturbance (at which point treatment must be withdrawn).

✚ warning: benzhexol hydrochloride should not be administered to patients who not only have tremor but distinct involuntary movements; it should be administered with caution to those with impaired kidney or liver function, cardiovascular disease, glaucoma, or urinary

B

retention. Withdrawal of treatment must be gradual. *Related articles:* ARTANE; BENTEX; BROFLEX.

benzocaine is a local ANAESTHETIC used in topical application for the relief of pain in the skin surface or mucous membranes, particularly in or around the mouth and throat, or (in combination with other drugs) in the ears. Administration is in various forms: as a cream, as anal suppositories, as an ointment, and as ear-drops.

- ● warning: prolonged use should be avoided; some patients experience sensitivity reactions.

benzodiazepines are a large group of drugs that have a marked effect upon the central nervous system. They increase the effectiveness of the inhibitory NEUROTRANSMITTER, GABA, in the central nervous system. The effect varies with different members of the group, however, and some are used primarily as SEDATIVES OF HYPNOTICS, whereas others are used more as ANXIOLYTICS, MUSCLE RELAXANTS OR ANTICONVULSANTS. Those that are used as hypnotics have virtually replaced the barbiturates, for the benzodiazepines are just as effective but are much safer in the event of an overdose, although some caution is necessary in treating patients who suffer from respiratory depression. There are now antagonists for reversing the effects of benzodiazepines (for instance at the end of operations): *see* FLUMAZENIL. It is now realized that serious dependence may result from continued usage, particularly with short-acting benzodiazepines, and that also there may be a paradoxical increase in hostility, paranoia and aggresion in those on longer-term treatment. Best-known and most-used benzodiazepines include diazepam (used particularly to control the convulsions of epilepsy or drug poisoning), nitrazepam (a widely used hypnotic) and lorazepam (an anxiolytic).

- ▲/● side-effects/warning: *see* ALPRAZOLAM; BROMAZEPAM; CHLORDIAZEPOXIDE; CLONAZEPAM; DIAZEPAM; FLUNITRAZEPAM; FLURAZEPAM; LOPRAZOLAM; LORAZEPAM; LORMETAZEPAM; MEDAZEPAM; OXAZEPAM; TEMAZEPAM.

benztropine mesylate is an ANTICHOLINERGIC agent employed in the treatment of some types of parkinsonism (*see* ANTI-PARKINSONIAN). It decreases rigidity and has a limited effect on tremors. The tendency to produce an excess of saliva is also reduced. (The drug also has the capacity to treat these conditions, in some cases, where they are produced by drugs.) It is thought to work by compensating for the lack of the neurotransmitter DOPAMINE in the brain, which is the major cause of such parkinsonian symptoms, and because it additionally has some sedative properties it is sometimes used in preference to the similar drug benzhexol hydrochloride. Administration – which may be in parallel with the administration of levodopa – is oral in the form of tablets, or by injection.

- ▲ side-effects: there may be drowsiness, dry mouth, dizziness and blurred vision, and/or gastrointestinal disturbances. Some patients experience sensitivity reactions.
- ● warning: benztropine mesylate should not be administered to patients who suffer not merely from tremor but from distinct

involuntary movements; it should be administered with caution to those with impaired kidney or liver function, cardiovascular disease, glaucoma, or urinary retention. Withdrawal of treatment must be gradual. *Related article:* COGENTIN.

benzydamine hydrochloride has ANALGESIC, local ANAESTHETIC and ANTI-INFLAMMATORY actions. It is used in topical application as a cream to relieve muscle or joint pain, or as a liquid mouthwash or spray to relieve the pain of mouth ulcers and other sores or inflammations in the mouth and throat. Some patients prefer to use the liquid in dilute form.

▲ side-effects: some patients experience a stinging sensation or numbness on initial application.

✚ warning: benzydamine is not recommended for continual use over more than 7 days. As a spray it is not suitable for children aged under 6 years; as a mouthwash it is not suitable for those aged under 13 years.

Berkolol (*Berk*) is a non-proprietary BETA-BLOCKER, available only on prescription, used to reduce frequency of migraine attacks. It may also be used to treat some of the manifestations of anxiety, e.g. rapid heart rate and tremor. Produced in the form of tablets (in four strengths), Berkolol is a preparation of the BETA-BLOCKER propranolol hydrochloride.

▲/✚ side-effects/warning: *see* PROPRANOLOL.

***beta-blockers** (beta-adrenoceptor blockers) are drugs that inhibit the action of the hormonal and NEUROTRANSMITTER substances ADRENALINE and NORADRENALINE in the body. These two catecholamines are involved in bodily response to stress: among other actions they speed the heart and constrict some blood vessels, so increasing blood pressure, suppress digestion and generally prepare the body for emergency action. They may also cause fine muscle tremor. Beta-blockers are administered so that the receptor sites that would normally react to the presence of the catecholamines remain comparatively inactivated. They may be useful in preventing some of the unpleasant manifestations of anxiety (*see* ANXIOLYTIC), such as a fast heart beat and fine muscle tremor. They may also be useful in the prophylactic treatment of migraine. Care must be taken in prescribing for patients with disorders of the respiratory tract, because their use may induce asthma attacks. The best-known and most-used beta-blocker for these purposes is propranolol.

▲/✚ side-effects/warning: *see* METOPROLOL; NADOLOL; OXPRENOLOL; PROPRANOLOL; TIMOLOL.

betahistine hydrochloride is an ANTINAUSEANT drug used specifically to treat the vertigo and nausea associated with Ménière's disease (which also causes constant noises in the ears). Administration is oral in the form of tablets.

▲ side-effects: sometimes the drug, while helping to relieve vertigo, actually causes nausea; some patients experience a headache; rarely, there may be a rash.

✚ warning: betahistine hydrochloride should not be administered to patients who suffer from abnormal secretion from the tumours of adrenal gland tissue (phaeo-chromocytoma); it should be administered with caution to those who suffer from asthma

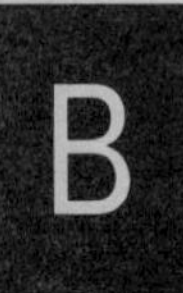

or peptic ulcer.
Related article: SERC.

Betaloc (*Astra*) is a proprietary preparation of the BETA-BLOCKER metoprolol tartrate, available only on prescription, used occasionally in the prevention of migraine attacks. Produced in a standard form of tablets (in two strengths), a sustained-release form ('Durules') is also available (under the trade name Betaloc-SA) tablets. None of these is recommended for children.
▲/⬢ side-effects/warning: *see* METOPROLOL.

Betim (*Burgess*) is a proprietary BETA-BLOCKER, occasionally used prophylactically to reduce the frequency of migraine attacks. Produced in the form of tablets, Betim represents a preparation of timolol maleate. It is not recommended for children.
▲/⬢ side-effects/warning: *see* TIMOLOL.

Biorphen (*Bio-Medical*) is a proprietary ANTICHOLINERGIC drug, available only on prescription, used to relieve some of the symptoms of parkinsonism, especially muscle rigidity and the tendency to produce an excess of saliva (*see* ANTIPARKINSONIAN). The drug also has the capacity to treat these conditions in some cases where they are produced by drugs. It is thought to work by compensating for the lack of the neurotransmitter DOPAMINE in the brain that is the major cause of such parkinsonian symptoms. Produced in the form of a sugar-free elixir, Biorphen represents a preparation of orphenadrine hydrochloride. Counselling of patients is advised.
▲/⬢ side-effects/warning: *see* ORPHENADRINE HYDROCHLORIDE.

biperiden lactate is an ANTICHOLINERGIC agent employed in the treatment of some types of parkinsonism (*see* ANTIPARKINSONIAN). It decreases rigidity and has a limited effect on tremors. The tendency to produce an excess of saliva is also reduced. (The drug also has the capacity to treat these conditions in some cases where they are produced by drugs.) It is thought to work by compensating for the lack of the neurotransmitter DOPAMINE in the brain that is the major cause of such parkinsonian symptoms, and because it additionally has some SEDATIVE properties it is sometimes used in preference to the similar drug benzhexol hydrochloride. Administration – which may be in parallel with the administration of other drugs used to relieve parkinsonism – is oral in the form of tablets, or by injection.
▲ side-effects: there may be drowsiness, dry mouth, dizziness and blurred vision, and/or gastrointestinal disturbances. Some patients experience sensitivity reactions.
⬢ warning: biperiden should be administered only to patients with mild tremor and rigidity; it should be administered with caution to those with impaired kidney or liver function, cardiovascular disease, glaucoma, or urinary retention. Withdrawal of treatment must be gradual.
Related article: AKINETON.

Bolvidon (*Organon*) is a proprietary ANTIDEPRESSANT, available only on prescription, used to treat depressive illness especially where sedation is needed. Produced in the form of tablets (in three strengths), Bolvidon is a preparation of mianserin hydrochloride. It is not recommended for children.
▲/⬢ side-effects/warning: *see* MIANSERIN.

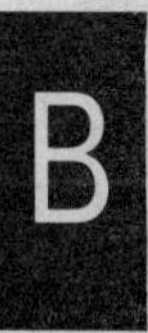

Brietal Sodium (*Lilly*) is a proprietary preparation of the short-acting general ANAESTHETIC methohexitone, in the form of methohexitone sodium. It is used mainly for the initial induction of anaesthesia or for short, minor operations. Available only on prescription, Brietal Sodium is produced in vials for intravenous injection (in three strengths).
▲/♦ side-effects/warning: *see* METHOHEXITONE SODIUM.

Brocadopa (*Brocades*) is a proprietary form of the drug levodopa, used to treat parkinsonism (*see* ANTIPARKINSONIAN). It is particularly good at relieving the rigidity and slowness of movement associated with the disease, although it does not always improve the tremor. Levodopa is converted inside the body to the neurotransmitter DOPAMINE – and it is the lack of dopamine in the brain that it is thought levodopa compensates for. It is produced in the form of capsules (in three strengths).
▲/♦ side-effects/warning: *see* LEVODOPA.

Broflex (*Bio-Medical*) is a proprietary preparation of the drug benzhexol hydrochloride, available only on prescription, used to relieve some of the symptoms of parkinsonism specifically the overall rigidity of the posture, and the tendency to produce an excess of saliva. The drug also has the capacity to treat these conditions in some cases where they are produced by drugs (*see* ANTIPARKINSONIAN). It is thought to work by compensating for the lack of the neurotransmitter DOPAMINE in the brain, which is the major cause of such parkinsonian symptoms. Broflex is produced in the form of a syrup for dilution (the potency of the syrup once diluted is retained for 14 days), to be taken before or after food; counselling of patients is advised. Broflex is not recommended for children.
▲/♦ side-effects/warning: *see* BENZHEXOL HYDROCHLORIDE.

bromazepam is an ANXIOLYTIC drug, one of the BENZODIAZEPINES used to treat anxiety in the short term. Administration is oral in the form of tablets. It is not recommended for children.
▲ side-effects: there may be drowsiness, unsteadiness, confusion, headache, and shallow breathing; hypersensitivity reactions may occur.
♦ warning: bromazepam may reduce a patient's concentration and speed of movement or thought; it may also enhance the effects of alcohol consumption. Prolonged use or abrupt withdrawal of treatment should be avoided. It should be administered with caution to patients with respiratory difficulties, or kidney or liver disease; who are in the last stages of pregnancy; or who are elderly or debilitated.
Related article: LEXOTAN.

bromocriptine is a drug used to treat certain hormonal disorders and parkinsonism, but not the parkinsonian symptoms caused by certain drug therapies (*see* ANTIPARKINSONIAN). It works by stimulating the DOPAMINE receptors in the brain as if the neurotransmitter dopamine was present in the correct amount. In this it is slightly different from the more commonly used treatment for Parkinson's disease, levodopa, which actually is converted to dopamine in the body. It is thus particularly useful in the treatment of patients who for one reason or another cannot tolerate levodopa. Occasionally,

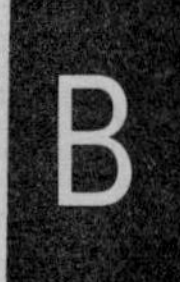

the two drugs are combined. However, bromocriptine is also used to treat delayed puberty caused by hormonal insufficiency, to relieve certain menstrual disorders, or to treat female infertility caused by excessive secretion of prolactin from the pituitary gland. Administration of bromocriptine is oral in the form of tablets and capsules.

▲ side-effects: there may be nausea, vomiting, headache, dizziness especially on rising from sitting or lying down (because of reduced blood pressure), and drowsiness. High dosage may cause hallucinations, a state of confusion, and leg cramps.

● warning: full, regular monitoring of various body systems is essential during treatment, particularly to check on whether there is pituitary enlargement.

Related article: PARLODEL.

Brompton Cocktails are various compound narcotic ANALGESIC elixirs containing MORPHINE or its derivatives, such as DIAMORPHINE (better known as heroin) and COCAINE). They were once widely used for the relief of severe pain during the final stages of terminal disease; now, however, preparations of only one narcotic analgesic or another are preferred.

Brufen (*Boots*) is a proprietary, non-steroidal, non-narcotic ANALGESIC that has valuable additional ANTI-INFLAMMATORY properties. Available only on prescription, Brufen is used to relieve pain – particularly the pain of rheumatic disease and other musculo-skeletal disorders – and is produced in the form of tablets (in three strengths) and as a syrup for dilution (the potency of the syrup once dilute is retained for 14 days) as a preparation of ibuprofen.

▲/● side-effects/warning: *see* IBUPROFEN.

Buccasten (*R & C*) is a proprietary form of the ANTI-EMETIC drug prochlorperazine. Available on prescription in the form of tablets, which are placed between the gum and upper lip, and left to dissolve.

▲/● side-effects/warning: *see* PROCHLORPERAZINE.

bupivacaine hydrochloride is a long-acting local ANAESTHETIC related to lignocaine, but is more potent and has greater duration of action. It is often administered by epidural injection via the spinal membranes (particularly to relieve pain during labour).

▲ side-effects: there may be slow heart rate and low blood pressure (hypotension), which may in high dosage tend towards cardiac arrest. Some patients enter states of euphoria, agitation or respiratory depression.

● warning: bupivacaine hydrochloride should not be administered to patients who suffer from the neural disorder myasthenia gravis or from heart block, or who are suffering from an insufficient supply of blood (as in shock); it should be administered with caution to those with impaired heart or liver function, or epilepsy. Dosage should be reduced for the elderly or debilitated. Facilities for emergency cardio-respiratory resuscitation should be on hand during treatment.

buprenorphine is a narcotic ANALGESIC that is long-acting and is used to treat moderate to severe levels of pain. Its effects last much longer than morphine, with a single sublingual dose lasting up to 12 hours. Although it is

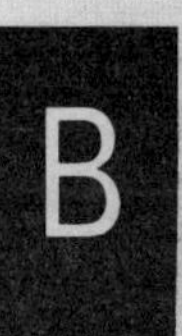

thought not to be as seriously addictive as morphine, it is on the Controlled Drugs list. Since it has some OPIATE antagonist properties it may be unwise to use in combination with other narcotic analgesics and can precipitate mild withdrawal symptoms in those habituated to, for instance, morphine or diamorphine. Its effects are not fully reversed by the usual OPIATE antagonist, naloxone. Administration is oral in the form of tablets placed sublingually, or by intramuscular or slow intravenous injection.

▲ side-effects: nausea, vomiting, dizziness, sweating and drowsiness are fairly common. There may be hypotension, mood changes and other side-effects. Rarely, there may be shallow breathing.

● warning: buprenorphine should not be administered to patients who suffer from head injury or increased intracranial pressure; it should be administered with caution to those with impaired kidney or liver function, asthma, depressed respiration, insufficient secretion of thyroid hormones (hypothyroidism) or low blood pressure (hypotension), or who are pregnant or lactating. Dosage should be reduced for the elderly or debilitated. It may precipitate withdrawal symptoms if given with other narcotic analgesics, and naloxone may not fully reverse its effects.
Related article: TEMGESIC.

buspirone hydrochloride is an ANXIOLYTIC drug usd for the short-term treatment of anxiety. It is a new drug and its mode of action and addictive liability is not yet established. Available on prescription in the form of tablets.

▲ side-effects: the effects of alcohol may be enhanced, and driving ability may be impaired. It may cause headache, nervousness, dizziness, nausea, excitment and light-headedness. Occasionally there may be chest pains, confusion, dry mouth, sweating, fatigue, and palpitations.

● warning: buspirone hydrochloride should not be administered to patients with severe liver or kidney damage, or who are pregnant, lactating, or are epipleptic.
Related article: BUSPAR.

Buspar (*Bristol-Myers*) is a proprietary form of the new ANXIOLYTIC drug buspirone hydrochloride. Available on prescription in the form of tablets in two strengths.

▲/● side-effects/warning: *see* BUSPIRONE HYDROCHLORIDE.

Butacote (*Geigy*) is a proprietary, ANTI-INFLAMMATORY, non-narcotic ANALGESIC, available only on prescription under specialized hospital care. It is used to treat rheumatic disease of the type that effects the spine (ankylosing spondylitis). Produced in the form of tablets (in two strengths), Butacote is a preparation of phenylbutazone.

▲/● side-effects/warning: *see* PHENYLBUTAZONE.

Butazone (*DDSA Pharmaceuticals*) is a proprietary, ANTI-INFLAMMATORY, non-narcotic ANALGESIC drug, available only on prescription in hospitals, used to treat rheumatic disease involving especially the spine. Produced in the form of tablets (in two strengths), Butazone represents a preparation of phenylbutazone.

▲/● side-effects/warning: *see* PHENYLBUTAZONE.

B

butobarbitone is a BARBITURATE used only when absolutely necessary as a HYPNOTIC, to treat severe and intractable insomnia. Administration is oral in the form of tablets – the proprietary preparation is on the controlled drugs list – to be taken about half an hour before retiring.

▲ side-effects: concentration and the speed of movement and thought are affected. There may be drowsiness, dizziness and shallow breathing, with headache. Some patients experience hypersensitivity reactions. (The drug enhances the effects of alcohol consumption.)

● warning: butobarbitone should not be administered to patients whose insomnia is caused by pain, who suffer from porphyria, who are pregnant or lactating, who are elderly or debilitated, or who have a history of drug (including alcohol) abuse. It should be administered with caution to those who suffer from kidney, liver or lung disease. Use of the drug should be avoided as far as possible. Repeated doses are cumulative in effect, and may lead to real sedation; abrupt withdrawal of treatment, on the other hand, may cause serious withdrawal symptoms. Tolerance and dependence occur readily.

Related article: SONERYL.

butriptyline is a tricyclic ANTIDEPRESSANT drug that also has some sedative properties, used to treat depressive illness, especially where there is also some degree of anxiety. Administration of butriptyline is oral in the form of tablets.

▲ side-effects: common effects include sedation (affecting driving ability), dry mouth, and blurred vision; there may also be difficulty in urinating, sweating, and irregular heartbeat, behavioural disturbances, a rash, a state of confusion, and/or a loss of libido. Rarely, there are also blood disorders.

● warning: butriptyline should not be administered to patients who suffer from heart disease or psychosis; it should be administered with caution to those with diabetes, epilepsy, liver or thyroid disease, glaucoma, or urinary retention; or who are pregnant or lactating. Withdrawal of treatment must be gradual.

Related article: EVADYNE.

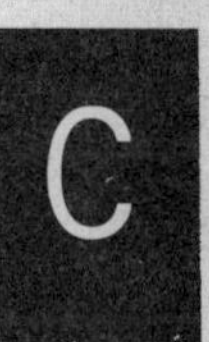

Cafadol (*Typharm*) is a non-prescription, non-narcotic compound ANALGESIC, which is not available from the National Health Service. Used for mild pain, it is produced in the form of tablets. Cafadol is a compound of paracetamol and caffeine.
▲/ ✚ side-effects/warning: *see* CAFFEINE; PARACETAMOL.

Cafergot (*Sandoz*) is a proprietary ANALGESIC, available only on prescription, used to treat migraine. Produced in the form of tablets and suppositories, Cafergot is a compound of caffeine and ergotamine tartrate.
▲/ ✚ side-effects/warning: *see* CAFFEINE; ERGOTAMINE TARTRATE.

caffeine is a weak STIMULANT. Present in both tea and coffee, it is included in many ANALGESIC preparations, often to increase absorption. In the form of caffeine sodium benzoate, it is used as a cardiac stimulant.
▲ side-effects: excessive doses may cause headache, either directly or on withdrawal, anxiety, or gastrointestinal upset.
✚ warning: caffeine should not be taken simultaneously with aspirin, or increased gastric irritation may occur.

Calpol (*Calmic*) is a proprietary form of the non-narcotic ANALGESIC paracetamol. It is produced in the form of a suspension in two strengths: the weaker (non-prescription) is produced under the name Calpol Infant, which is also available in a sugar-free form; the stronger (not available from the National Health Service) under the name Calpol Six Plus.
▲/ ✚ side-effects/warning: *see* PARACETAMOL.

Camcolit (*Norgine*) is a proprietary drug for the treament of manic-depressive illness, available only on prescription. Produced in the form of tablets (in two strengths), Camcolit is a preparation of lithium carbonate. It is not recommended for children.
▲/ ✚ side-effects/warning: *see* LITHIUM.

cannabis is one name for a drug prepared from the Indian hemp plant Cannabis sativa: other names include bhang, dagga, hashish, marijuana and pot. Its use seems of little therapeutic value, and its social use is illegal although fairly widespread. (It may be prescribed only under licence from the Home Secretary.) A synthetic cannabinoid, NABILONE, is used in cancer chemotherapy to reduce nausea and vomiting.
▲ side-effects: smoked or ingested, cannabis is a psychedelic, causing comparatively mild hallucinations with euphoria, heightening awareness and particularly affecting the sense of time. Withdrawal symptoms are rare, but use tends to increase tolerance.
✚ warning: prolonged use has been suggested to result in a degree of brain damage, and is thought by some to lead a user to experiment with addictive 'hard' drugs, although it is difficult to test either theory.

Caprin (*Sinclair*) is a proprietary, non-prescription preparation of the non-narcotic ANALGESIC aspirin, used particularly to treat headache and rheumatic conditions. Produced in the form of sustained-release tablets, Caprin is not recommended for children aged under 12 years.
▲/ ✚ side-effects/warning: *see* ASPIRIN.

carbamazepine is an ANTICONVULSANT drug used, sometimes in combination with

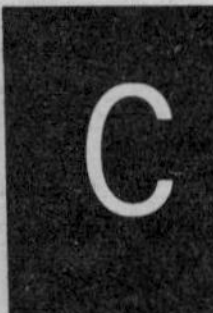

other drugs, particularly to treat various forms of 'cortical' epilepsy including temporal lobe and grand mal epilepsy. In smaller doses it is effective in reducing attacks of trigeminal neuralgia (a searing pain in paroxysms along the trigeminal nerve in the face) or the neural disorders that may accompany diabetes mellitus, again on a maintenance basis. Surprisingly, it is sometimes used in the treatment of diabetes insipidus. Carbamazepine may also be used for treating manic-depressive illness unresponsive to lithium.

▲ side-effects: there may be blurring of vision and unsteadiness; high dosage may cause severe dizziness. Sometimes there are gastrointestinal disturbances; occasionally there is a rash.

● warning: carbamazepine should not be administered to patients who suffer from certain heart defects or porphyria, or to those using or having recently used any of the MAO INHIBITOR drugs; it should be administered with caution to those who suffer from impaired function of the liver or glaucoma, or who are lactating. Dosage should begin at a minimum level and be adjusted upwards for optimum effect. Blood monitoring is essential if high doses are administered.

Related article: TEGRETOL.

carbidopa is a drug administered in combination with levodopa to treat parkinsonism, but not the parkinsonian symptoms induced by other drugs (*see* ANTIPARKINSONIAN). It is levodopa that actually has the therapeutic effect. Carbidopa inhibits the breakdown of levodopa (to DOPAMINE) in the body before it reaches the brain, where it carries out its function. The presence of carbidopa allows the dose of levodopa to be at a minimum, thus also minimizing potentially severe side-effects, and speeds the therapeutic response. Administration of carbidopa and levodopa is in the form of single compound tablets.

▲/● side-effects/warning: *see* LEVODOPA.

Related article: SINEMET.

carbinoxamine is a short-acting ANTIHISTAMINE that is an anti-allergic constituent in one or two cough linctuses and, because it also has mild ANTINAUSEANT properties, is also found in some proprietary preparations to prevent travel sickness.

Cesamet (*Lilly*) is a proprietary ANTI-EMETIC, available only on prescription, used to treat nausea in patients undergoing chemotherapy in the treatment of cancer. Produced in the form of capsules, Cesamet's active constituent is the synthetic cannabinoid nabilone. It is not recommended for children.

▲/● side-effects/warning: *see* NABILONE.

Chloractil (*DDSA Pharmaceuticals*) is a proprietary preparation of the PHENOTHIAZINE drug chlorpromazine hydrochloride, used primarily as a major TRANQUILLIZER in patients who are undergoing severe behavioural disturbances, or who are psychotic (*see* ANTIPSYCHOTIC) particularly schizophrenic. It may also be used to treat severe anxiety, or as an ANTI-EMETIC and SEDATIVE in terminal cancer. Available only on prescription, Chloractil is produced in the form of tablets (in three strengths).

▲/● side-effects/warning: *see* CHLORPROMAZINE.

chloral hydrate is a water-soluble HYPNOTIC, which is rapid-acting. It is useful in inducing sleep in

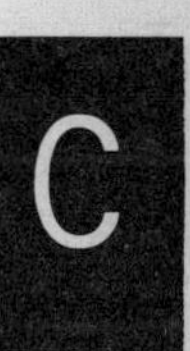

children or elderly patients, although the drug must be administered in very mild solution in order to minimize gastric irritation. Administration is thus usually oral, although it can alternatively be rectal. Overdosage results in toxic effects; prolonged use may lead to dependence (addiction).

▲ side-effects: concentration and speed of thought and movement are affected. There is often drowsiness and dizziness, with dry mouth. Sensitivity reactions are also fairly common, especially in the form of rashes. Susceptible patients may experience excitement or confusion.

● warning: chloral hydrate should not be administered to patients with severe heart disease, inflammation of the stomach, or impaired function of the liver or kidneys. It should be administered with caution to those with lung disease and respiratory depression, who are pregnant or lactating, who are elderly or debilitated, or who have a history of drug abuse. Contact with skin or mucous membranes should be avoided.
Related article: NOCTEC.

chlordiazepoxide is an ANXIOLYTIC drug, one of the earliest of the BENZODIAZEPINES, used to treat anxiety in the short-term, and to assist in the treatment of acute alcohol withdrawal symptoms. It may also be used as a SKELETAL MUSCLE RELAXANT. Continued use results in tolerance and may lead to dependence (addiction). Administration is oral in the form of capsules and tablets.

▲ side-effects: concentration and speed of thought and movement may be affected; the effects of alcohol consumption may also be enhanced. Confusion, unsteadiness, headache, shallow breathing and hypersensitivity reactions may occur. Dependence may result with long-term use.

● warning: chlordiazepoxide should be administered with caution to patients with respiratory difficulties, glaucoma, or kidney or liver impairment; who are in the last stages of pregnancy; or who are elderly, debilitated, or have a history of drug abuse. Prolonged use or abrupt withdrawal of treatment should be avoided.
Related articles: LIBRIUM; TROPIUM.

chlormethiazole is a HYPNOTIC drug that also has ANTI-CONVULSANT properties. It is useful in treating severe insomnia, status epilepticus, and for quieting agitated elderly patients, and it is also used under strict medical supervision in the treatment of alcohol withdrawal. Tolerance and dependence may occur with long-term use. Administration (in the form of chlormethiazole edisylate) is oral as capsules or dilute syrup, or by injection or infusion.

▲ side-effects: there may be headache, sneezing and gastrointestinal disturbance. High dosage by intravenous infusion may cause depressed breathing and reduced heart rate, and presents a risk of thrombophlebitis.

● warning: chlormethiazole should be administered with caution to patients with restricted breathing, or impaired liver or kidney function, who are pregnant or lactating, who are elderly or debilitated, or who have a history of drug abuse. Prolonged use should be avoided; withdrawal of

C

treatment should be gradual.
Related article: HEMINEVRIN.

chlormezanone is an ANXIOLYTIC drug that has HYPNOTIC properties and may be tried as a SKELETAL MUSCLE RELAXANT. It is thus used to treat anxiety and tension in the short term (including pre-menstrual syndrome), to induce sleep and to relieve muscle spasm. Administration is oral in the form of tablets.

▲ side-effects: concentration and speed of thought and movement may be affected; the effects of alcohol consumption may also be enhanced. There may be drowsiness, dizziness, headache, dry mouth and shallow breathing; hypersensitivity reactions may occur.

● warning: chlormezanone should be administered with caution to patients with respiratory difficulties, closed angle glaucoma, or kidney or liver disease; who are in the last stages of pregnancy; or who are elderly or debilitated. Prolonged use or abrupt withdrawal of treatment should be avoided.
Related article: TRANCOPAL.

chlorpromazine is the classic PHENOTHIAZINE type ANTIPSYCHOTIC drug used as a major TRANQUILLIZER for patients suffering from schizophrenia and other psychoses. The drug may also be used in the short-term to treat severe anxiety, to soothe patients who are dying, as a premedication prior to surgery, and to remedy an intractable hiccup. It may also be used to relieve nausea and vertigo caused by disorders in the middle or inner ear. Administration (as chlorpromazine hydrochloride) is oral in the form of tablets or an elixir, as anal suppositories, or by intramuscular injection.

▲ side-effects: concentration and speed of thought and movement are affected; the effects of alcohol consumption are enhanced. High doses may cause extrapyramidal movement disorders. Muscle spasms (dystonias) and Parkinsonian-like rigidity, tremor and slow movement may occur. Prolonged use may also cause abnormal compulsive movements of the hands, face and head (tardive dyskinesias). There may be dry mouth and blocked nose, constipation and difficulty in urinating, and blurred vision; menstrual disturbances in women or impotence in men may occur, with weight gain; there may be sensitivity reactions. Some patients feel cold and depressed, and tend to suffer from poor sleep patterns. Blood pressure may be low and the heartbeat irregular. Prolonged high dosage may cause opacity in the cornea and lens of the eyes, and a purple pigmentation of the skin. Treatment by intramuscular injection may be painful.

● warning: chlorpromazine hydrochloride should not be administered to patients with certain forms of glaucoma, whose blood-cell formation by the bone-marrow is reduced, or who are taking drugs that depress certain centres of the brain and spinal cord. It should be administered with caution to those with lung disease, cardiovascular disease, epilepsy, parkinsonism, abnormal secretion by the adrenal glands, impaired liver or kidney function, undersecretion of thyroid hormones (hypothyroidism), enlargement of the prostate gland, or any form of acute

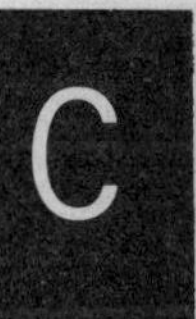

infection; who are pregnant or lactating; or who are elderly. Prolonged use requires regular checks on eye function and skin pigmentation. Withdrawal of treatment should be gradual. *Related articles:* CHLORACTIL; LARGACTIL.

choline magnesium trisalicylate is an non-narcotic ANALGESIC with ANTI-INFLAMMATORY properties very similar to aspirin, used to treat the pain and inflammation of rheumatic disease and other musculo-skeletal disorders. Administration is oral in the form of tablets.
▲ side-effects: there may be gastrointestinal problems involving ulceration or bleeding, nausea, and disturbances in hearing and in vision; some patients experience serious sensitivity reactions.
✚ warning: choline magnesium trisalicylate should not be administered to patients who are aged under 12 years, or who have peptic ulcers; it should be administered with caution to those with impaired liver or kidney function, dehydration or any form of allergy, who are pregnant or lactating, who are elderly, or who are already taking oral anticoagulant drugs. *Related article:* TRILISATE.

choline salicylate is a mild ANALGESIC and local ANAESTHETIC, which is used primarily in topical application in the mouth or in the ears. In the mouth it may be used to relieve the pain of teething, of aphthous ulcers or of minor scratches. Administration is in the form of an oral gel or ear-drops.
✚ warning: prolonged treatment may result in salicylate poisoning. *Related articles:* AUDAX; TEEJEL.

cinnarizine is an ANTIHISTAMINE used primarily as an ANTI-EMETIC in the treatment or prevention of motion sickness and vomiting caused by disorders of the middle or inner ear, e.g. Ménière's disease. Administration is oral in the form of tablets. Not recommended for children under 6 years.
▲ side-effects: concentration and speed of thought and movement may be affected. There is commonly drowsiness and dry mouth; there may also be headache, blurred vision and gastrointestinal disturbances.
✚ warning: cinnarizine should be administered with caution to patients with epilepsy, liver disease, glaucoma or enlargement of the prostate gland. Drowsiness may be increased by alcohol consumption. *Related article:* MARZINE RF; STUGERON.

Citanest (*Astra*) is a proprietary local ANAESTHETIC, available only on prescription. Produced in vials (in two strengths) for injection, Citanest is a preparation of prilocaine hydrochloride.
▲/✚ side-effects/warning: *see* PRILOCAINE.

Citanest with Octapressin (*Astra*) is a proprietary local ANAESTHETIC, available only on prescription, used as a dental anaesthetic and as premedication before surgery. Produced in cartridges and self-aspirating cartridges for injection (in two strengths), Citanest with Octapressin contains prilocaine hydrochloride and the VASOCONSTRICTOR felypressin.
▲/✚ side-effects/warning: *see* PRILOCAINE.

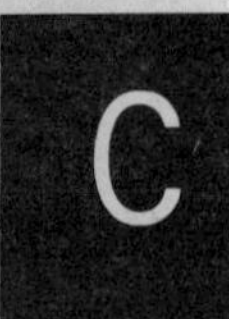

Clairvan (*Sinclair*) is a proprietary respiratory stimulant, available only on prescription, used to treat patients about to lapse into unconsciousness or coma and who are unable, for one reason or another, to tolerate the more usual forms of ventilatory support. Produced in the form of a solution to be taken orally, and in ampoules for injection, Clairvan's active constituent is ethamivan.
▲/✚ side-effects/warning: *see* ETHAMIVAN.

Clazaril (*Sandoz*) is an ANTIPSYCHOTIC, a proprietary form of clozapine available only on prescription in the form of tablets (in two strengths). Subject to special monitoring for potentially severe effects on the blood.
▲/✚ side-effects/warning: *see* CLOZAPINE.

Clinoril (*Merck, Sharp & Dohme*) is a proprietary, non-steroidal, anti-inflammatory, non-narcotic ANALGESIC, available only on prescription, used to treat rheumatic conditions and acute gout. Produced in the form of tablets (in two strengths), Clinoril is a preparation of sulindac.
▲/✚ side-effects/warning: *see* SULINDAC.

clobazam is an ANXIOLYTIC drug, one of the BENZODIAZEPINES, used to treat anxiety in the short term, and sometimes to assist in the treatment of some forms of epilepsy. Administration is oral in the form of capsules.
▲ side-effects: concentration and speed of thought and movement may be affected; the effects of alcohol consumption may be enhanced.
✚ warning: clobazam should be administered with caution to patients with depressed respiration. Prolonged use and abrupt withdrawal of treatment should be avoided.
Related article: FRISIUM.

clomipramine hydrochloride is a tricyclic ANTIDEPRESSANT drug that has mild sedative properties. It is used primarily to treat depressive illness, but can be used to assist in treating phobic or obsessional states, and to try to reduce the incidence of cataplexy in narcoleptic patients. Administration is oral in the form of capsules, sustained-release tablets, and a dilute syrup, or by injection.
▲ side-effects: sedation that may affect driving ability; there is also dry mouth. There may also be blurred vision, difficulty in urinating, sweating, and irregular heartbeat, behavioural disturbances, a rash, a state of confusion, and/or a loss of libido. Rarely, there are also blood disorders.
✚ warning: clomipramine hydrochloride should not be administered to patients with heart disease; it should be administered with caution to those with diabetes, epilepsy, liver or thyroid disease, glaucoma, or urinary retention; or who are pregnant or lactating. Withdrawal of treatment must be gradual.
Related article: ANAFRANIL.

clonazepam is a BENZODIAZEPINE, but it is used as an ANTICONVULSANT drug in the treatment of all forms of epilepsy. Tolerance to its anti-epileptic effects occurs over a period of weeks. Administration is oral in the form of tablets.
▲ side-effects: sedation that may affect driving ability; in susceptible patients the degree of sedation may be marked. It also enhances the effects of alcohol consumption. There may also be dizziness, fatigue and muscular weakness. Again

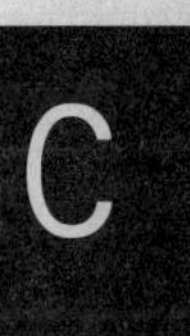

in susceptible patients, there may be mood changes.
- ✚ warning: clonazepam should be administered with caution to patients who are lactating. The drug is more sedative than most drugs used to treat epilepsy.
Related article: RIVOTRIL.

clonidine hydrochloride is primarily an antihypertensive drug used to treat moderate to severe high blood pressure (hypertension). Although controversial, use of the drug has also been extended to assisting in the prevention of migraine attacks. Administration is oral in the form of tablets and sustained-release capsules, or by injection.
- ▲ side-effects: there is sedation and dry mouth; there may also be fluid retention (oedema), a reduced heart rate, and depression.
- ✚ warning: clonidine hydrochloride should not be administered to patients who have a history of depression. Treatment must be withdrawn gradually (in order to avoid a hypertensive crisis).

Clopenthixol is an alternative proprietary name for the powerful ANTIPSYCHOTIC drug zuclopenthixol.
see ZUCLOPENTHIXOL.

Clopixol (*Lundbeck*) is a proprietary ANTIPSYCHOTIC drug, available only on prescription, used to treat and restrain psychotic patients, particularly more aggressive or agitated schizophrenics. Clopixol is produced in several forms. Preparations of zuclopenthixol dihydrochloride are available as tablets (in three strengths) called Clopixol; zuclopenthixol decanoate is prepared as oily depot injections in two strengths, the weaker called Clopixol and the stronger called Clopixol Conc.); and of zuclopenthixol acetate as an oily depot injection called Clopixol Acuphase. The preparations differ in their duration of action and may be used according to the length of treatment intended.
- ▲/✚ side-effects/warning: *see* ZUCLOPENTHIXOL.

clorazepate dipotassium is an ANXIOLYTIC drug, one of the BENZODIAZEPINES, used to treat anxiety in the short term. Administration is oral in the form of capsules.
- ▲ side-effects: drowsiness affecting concentration and speed of thought and movement; the effects of alcohol consumption may be enhanced. Unsteadiness of gait in the elderly. Dependence may occur with prolonged use.
- ✚ warning: clorazepate dipotassium should not be administered to patients with depressed respiration; it should be administered with caution to those with psychosis or phobic states. Prolonged use and abrupt withdrawal of treatment should be avoided.
Related article: TRANXENE.

clozapine is an ANTIPSYCHOTIC drug used for the treatment of schizophrenia in patients who do not respond to, or who can not tolerate more standard antipsychotics. It is less likely to cause extrapyramidal symptoms, but it can cause serious blood disorders (leucocytopenia and agranulocytosis), its use is therefore restricted to use in patients registered with the Sandoz Clozaril Patient Monitoring Service. It is available only on prescription, and in the form of tablets.
- ▲ side-effects: potentially very serious effects on the blood (agranulocytosis and

C

neutropenia), possible extrapyramidal symptoms, over salivation after initial dry mouth, tachycardia (speeding of the heart), postural hypotension (fall in blood pressure on standing up), gastrointestinal disturbances, difficulties in focussing of the eyes, changes in heart rhythms; and more rarely a number of other disturbances.

✚ warning: because of its effects on the blood (especially depressing the white cell count) this drug may only be used on registration with, and concurrent monitoring by, the special patient monitoring service. Any infections in the patient should be reported. Use of clozapine should be avoided in children, those with liver or kidney function impairment, epilepsy, cardiovascular disorders, in those with enlarged prostate gland, glaucoma, and certain gastrointestinal disorders. It should not be used in patients with a history of drug-induced neutropenia (lowered neutrophil white blood cell count) or agranulocytosis (lowered blood platelet count); bone marrow disorders, alcohol or drug induced psychoses; breast feeding or pregnancy; severe depression of the central nervous system or coma.

Related articles: CLAZARIL; CLOZARIL.

Clozaril (*Sandoz*) is a proprietary form of the ANTIPSYCHOTIC drug clozapine. Available on prescription to treat schizophrenia in patients unresponsive or intolerant to other antipsychotics. Available in hospitals only in the form of tablets (in 2 strengths). Registration with the Sandoz Clozaril Patient Monitoring Service is required.

▲/✚ side-effects/warning: *see* CLOZAPINE.

co-beneldopa is a mixture of the ANTIPARKINSONIAN drug levodopa with the enzyme-inhibitor benserazide hydrochloride, which prevents the peripheral degradation of levodopa to dopamine and therefore allows more levodopa to reach the brain.

Related article: MADOPAR.

co-careldopa is a mixture of the ANTIPARKINSONIAN drug levodopa with the enzyme-inhibitor carbidopa. Carbidopa prevents the peripheral degradation of levodopa to dopamine and therefore allows more levodopa to reach the brain.

Related article: SINEMET.

cocaine is a central nervous system STIMULANT that rapidly causes dependence (addiction). Because of its toxicity it is rarely used now, and then only as a local ANAESTHETIC for topical application, particularly (as cocaine hydrochloride, with or without the atropine derivative homatropine) in eye-drops. Its use as an analgesic, and especially as a constituent in elixirs prescribed to treat pain in terminal care (including the BROMPTON COCKTAILS), is now virtually discontinued.

co-codamol is a compound ANALGESIC combining the OPIATE codeine phosphate with paracetamol in a ratio of 8:500 (mg). As a compound it forms a constituent in a large number of proprietary analgesic preparations.

▲/✚ side-effects/warning: *see* CODEINE PHOSPHATE; PARACETAMOL.

Related articles: PARACODAL; PARAKE; PANADEINE.

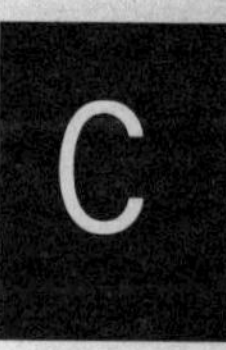

co-codaprin is a compound ANALGESIC combining the OPIATE codeine phosphate with aspirin in a ratio of 8:400 (mg). As a compound it forms a constituent in a number of proprietary analgesic preparations, but although it has the advantages of both drugs, it also has their disadvantages.

▲/ ✚ side-effects/warning: *see* ASPIRIN; CODEINE PHOSPHATE.
Related article: CODIS.

Codanin (*Whitehall Laboratories*) is a proprietary, non-prescription ANALGESIC produced in the form of tablets and as a powder. It is a preparation of codeine phosphate and paracetamol.

▲/ ✚ side-effects/warning: *see* CODEINE PHOSPHATE; PARACETAMOL.

codeine phosphate is an OPIATE, a narcotic ANALGESIC that also has the properties of a cough suppressant (ANTITUSSIVE). As an analgesic, codeine is a common, but often minor, constituent in non-proprietary and proprietary preparations to relieve pain (the majority of which are not available from the National Health Service), although some authorities dislike any combined form that contains codeine. Even more authorities disapprove of the drug's use as a cough suppressant. The drug also has the capacity to reduce intestinal motility (and so treat diarrhoea). Administration is oral or by injection.

▲ side-effects: tolerance occurs readily, although dependence (addiction) is relatively unusual. Constipation is common. There may be sedation and dizziness, especially following injection. The effects of alcohol consumption may be enhanced.

✚ warning: codeine phosphate should not be administered to patients who suffer from depressed breathing, or who are aged under 12 months.
Related articles: ANTOIN; CO-CODAMOL; CO-CODAPRIN; CODIS; DIMOTANE WITH CODEINE; FORMULIX; GALCODINE; HYPON; MEDOCODENE; MIGRALEVE; NEURODYNE; PANADEINE; PARACODOL; PARADEINE; PARAHYPON; PARAKE; PARAMOL; PARDALE; PHENSEDYL; PROPAIN; SOLPADEINE; SOLPADOL; TERCODA; TERPOIN; TYLEX; UNIFLU PLUS GREGOVITE; VEGANIN.

co-dergocrine mesylate is a VASODILATOR that affects the blood vessels of the brain. It is sometimes claimed to improve brain function, but clinical results of psychological tests during and following treatment have neither proved nor disproved that claim, and patients with senile dementia seem to derive little, if any, benefit. It is for the treatment of senile dementia that the drug has been most frequently prescribed.

▲ side-effects: there may be nausea and vomiting, flushing, a blocked nose, and a rash. Low blood pressure may cause dizziness on standing up from a lying or sitting position.

✚ warning: co-dergocrine mesylate should be administered with caution to patients who have a particularly slow heart rate.
Related article: HYDERGINE.

Codis (*Reckitt & Colman*) is a proprietary compound ANALGESIC, which is not available from the National Health Service. Used to relieve pain and high body temperature, and produced in the form of soluble (dispersible) tablets, Codis contains a combination of ASPIRIN with CODEINE PHOSPHATE (a combination itself known as co-

codaprin). It is not recommended for children.
▲/ ✚ side-effects/warning: *see* CO-CODAPRIN.

co-dydramol is a compound ANALGESIC, available on prescription, combining the NARCOTIC OPIATE dihydrocodeine with paracetamol in a ratio of 10:500 (mg). As a compound it forms a constituent of proprietary analgesic preparations, but although it has the advantages of both drugs, it also has the disadvantages. Since it contains a narcotic analgesic, dihydrocodeine is particularly dangerous in overdose, when it requires rapid hospitalization for the patient.
▲/ ✚ side-effects/warning: *see* DEXTROPROPOXYPHENE; PARACETAMOL.
Related article: COSALGESIC.

Cogentin (*Merck, Sharp & Dohme*) is a proprietary preparation of the ANTICHOLINERGIC drug benztropine mesylate, available only on prescription, used in the treatment of parkinsonism (*see* ANTIPARKINSONIAN) and to control tremors within drug-induced states. Produced in the form of tablets and in ampoules for injection, Cogentin is not recommended for children aged under 3 years.
▲/ ✚ side-effects/warning: *see* BENZTROPINE MESYLATE.

Coldrex (*Sterling Health*) is a proprietary, non-prescription cold relief preparation produced in the form of tablets and as a powder. It contains paracetamol, phenylephrine (to vasoconstrict the nasal membrane and so decrease nasal secretions) and ascorbic acid. The tablet formulation also contains the STIMULANT caffeine.
▲/ ✚ side-effects/warning: *see* CAFFEINE; PARACETAMOL; PHENYLEPHRINE.

Concordin (*Merck, Sharp & Dohme*) is a proprietary tricyclic ANTIDEPRESSANT available only on prescription, used to treat depressive illness, especially in apathetic or withdrawn patients. Produced in the form of tablets (in two strengths), Concordin is a preparation of protriptyline hydrochloride. It is not recommended for children.
▲/ ✚ side-effects/warning: *see* PROTRIPTYLINE.

Copholco (*Radiol Chemicals*) is a proprietary, non-prescription EXPECTORANT and cough mixture, which is not available from the National Health Service. Produced in the form of a linctus, Copholco is a preparation that includes the ANTITUSSIVE OPIATE pholcodine and menthol. It is not recommended for children aged under 5 years.
▲/ ✚ side-effects/warning: *see* PHOLCODINE.

co-proxamol is a compound ANALGESIC combining the NARCOTIC dextropropoxyphene with paracetamol in a ratio of 32.5:325 (mg). As a compound it forms a constituent in a number of proprietary analgesic preparations, but although it has the advantages of both drugs, it also has the disadvantages. Since it is a narcotic analgesic, dextropropoxyphene is particularly dangerous in overdose, when it requires rapid hospitalization for the subject.
▲/ ✚ side-effects/warning: *see* DEXTROPROPOXYPHENE; PARACETAMOL.
Related articles: COSALGESIC; DISTALGESIC; PAXALGESIC.

Corgard (*Squibb*) is a proprietary BETA-BLOCKER antihypertensive drug, available only on prescription, used to prevent migraine. Produced in the form of

tablets (in two strengths), Corgard is a preparation of nadolol. It is not recommended for children.
▲/♦ side-effects/warning: *see* NADOLOL.

Cosalgesic (*Cox*) is a proprietary ANALGESIC available only on prescription to private patients. Used to relieve pain anywhere in the body, and produced in the form of tablets, Cosalgesic is a preparation of the narcotic-like analgesic dextropropoxyphene together with paracetamol. (This compound combination is known as CO-PROXAMOL). It is not recommended for children.
▲/♦ side-effects/warning: see DEXTROPROPOXYPHENE; PARACETAMOL.

Cough Caps (*Beechams*) is a proprietary ANTITUSSIVE (cough suppressant) preparation available without prescription as sustained-release tablets. Its active principal agent is dextromethorphan.
▲/♦ side-effects/warning: *see* DEXTROMETHORPHAN.

cyclandelate is a VASODILATOR that specifically affects the blood vessels of the brain. It is sometimes claimed to improve brain function, but clinical results of psychological tests during and following treatment have neither proved nor disproved that claim, and patients suffering from senile dementia seem to derive little benefit if any. It is to assist in the treatment of senile dementia that the drug is most prescribed, although it can also be used to improve circulatory disorders of the limbs.
▲ side-effects: there may be nausea and flushing; high doses may cause dizziness.
♦ warning: cyclandelate should not be administered to patients who are suffering from brain injury.
Related article: CYCLOSPASMOL.

Cyclimorph (*Calmic*) is a proprietary form of the OPIATE NARCOTIC ANALGESIC morphine tartrate together with the ANTI-EMETIC ANTIHISTAMINE cyclizine tartrate, and is on the controlled drugs list. Used to treat moderate to severe pain, especially in serious conditions of fluid within the lungs, it is produced in ampoules (in two strengths, under the names Cyclimorph–10 and Cyclimorph–15) for injection. It is not recommended for children or for those in terminal care because of the sedative effects of cyclizine.
▲/♦ side-effects/warning: *see* CYCLIZINE; MORPHINE.

cyclizine is an ANTIHISTAMINE used primarily as an ANTI-EMETIC in the treatment or prevention of motion sickness and vomiting caused by disorders of the middle or inner ear. Administration (as cyclizine hydrochloride, cyclizine lactate or cyclizine tartrate) is oral in the form of tablets, or by injection.
▲ side-effects: concentration and speed of thought and movement may be affected. There is commonly drowsiness and dry mouth; there may also be headache, blurred vision and gastrointestinal disturbances.
♦ warning: cyclizine should be administered with caution to patients with heart failure, epilepsy, liver disease, glaucoma or enlargement of the prostate gland. Drowsiness may be increased by alcohol consumption.
Related articles: CYCLIMORPH; DICONAL; MIGRIL; VALOID.

cyclopropane is a gas used as an inhalant general ANAESTHETIC for both induction and maintenance

C

of general anaesthesia. It has some SKELETAL MUSCLE RELAXANT properties too, although in practice a muscle relaxant drug is usually administered simultaneously. However, it has the great disadvantage of being potentially explosive in air, and must be used via closed-circuit systems.

▲ side-effects: although recovery afterwards is rapid, there may be vomiting and agitation.

● warning: cyclopropane causes respiratory depression, and some form of assisted pulmonary ventilation may be necessary during anaesthesia.

Cyclospasmol (*Brocades*) is a proprietary, non-prescription VASODILATOR, used to improve blood circulation to the brain (suggested to be helpful in the treatment of senile dementia) and to the extremities. Produced in the form of capsules, as tablets and as a suspension for dilution (the potency of the suspension once dilute is retained for 14 days), Cyclospasmol is a preparation of cyclandelate.

▲/● side-effects/warning: *see* CYCLANDELATE.

cyproheptadine hydrochloride is an ANTIHISTAMINE sometimes used to treat migraine and – under medical supervision – as an appetite stimulant (especially in children). Administration is oral in the form of tablets or a dilute syrup.

▲ side-effects: there may be a sedative effect (or, in susceptible patients – especially children – excitement), a headache, and/or weight gain; some patients experience dry mouth, blurred vision, gastrointestinal disturbances and/or urinary retention.

● warning: cyproheptadine hydrochloride should be administered with caution to patients with epilepsy, glaucoma, liver disease or enlargement of the prostate gland

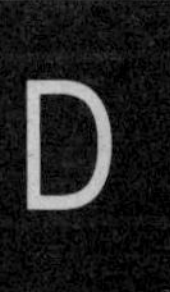

Dalmane (*Roche*) is a proprietary HYPNOTIC, available on prescription only to private patients, used to treat insomnia in cases where some degree of daytime sedation is acceptable. Produced in the form of capsules (in two strengths), Dalmane is a preparation of the long-acting BENZODIAZEPINE flurazepam.
▲/ ✚ side-effects/warning: *see* FLURAZEPAM.

Day Nurse (*Beecham Health Care*) is a proprietary, non-prescription cold-relief preparation produced in the form of tablets and as a syrup. It contains paracetamol, the VASOCONSTRICTOR decongestant phenyl-propanolamine and the ANTI-TUSSIVE dextromethorphan.
▲/ ✚ side-effects/warning: *see* PARACETAMOL; DEXTROMETHORPHAN.

Depixol (*Lundbeck*) is a proprietary ANTIPSYCHOTIC drug, available only on prescription, used to tranquillize patients suffering from psychosis (including schizophrenia), especially patients with forms of psychosis that render them apathetic and withdrawn. It may also be used in the short term to treat severe anxiety. Produced in the form of tablets, or in ampoules for injection (in two strengths, the stronger under the name Depixol Conc.), and as a depot injection. Depixol is a preparation of flupenthixol.
▲/ ✚ side-effects/warning: *see* FLUPENTHIXOL.

desipramine hydrochloride is a tricyclic ANTIDEPRESSANT drug type that has fewer sedative properties than many others. Used to treat depressive illness, it is thus suited more to the treatment of withdrawn and apathetic patients than to those who are agitated and restless. Administration is oral in the form of tablets.
▲ side-effects: common effects include sedation (affecting driving ability), dry mouth and blurred vision; there may also be difficulty in urinating, sweating and irregular heartbeat, behavioural disturbances, a rash, a state of confusion, and/or a loss of libido. Rarely, there are also blood disorders.
✚ warning: desipramine hydrochloride should not be administered to patients who suffer from heart disease or psychosis; it should be administered with caution to patients who suffer from diabetes, epilepsy, liver or thyroid disease, glaucoma or urinary retention; or who are pregnant or lactating. Withdrawal of treatment must be gradual.
Related article: PERTOFRAN.

dexamphetamine sulphate is an amphetamine, a powerful STIMULANT drug, used primarily to treat narcolepsy (a condition marked by irresistible attacks of sleep during the daytime), although it is sometimes also used under specialist supervision to treat children who are medically hyperactive. Tolerance and dependence (addiction) are major hazards. Administration is oral in the form of tablets and sustained-release capsules.
▲ side-effects: tolerance and dependence (addiction) occur readily. There may also be agitation, insomnia, headache and dizziness. Some patients experience heartbeat irregularities, dry mouth, diarrhoea or constipation. There may also be tremor and a personality change, night terrors, euphoria and anorexia. In children, drastic weight loss may be accompanied by

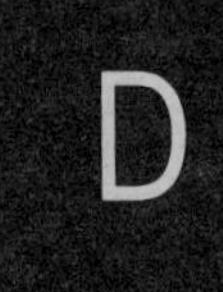

inhibition of growth. Overdoses may result in psychoses, convulsions, or even death.

- ● warning: dexamphetamine sulphate should not be administered to patients who suffer from severe hypertension, glaucoma, an excess of thyroid hormones in the bloodstream (thyrotoxicosis), or an unstable personality. It should also not be administered during pregnancy or lactation, or to patients with a history of drug abuse or extrapyramidal disorders. Care must be taken when prescribing to those with mild hypertension. Growth in children should be monitored and abrupt withdrawal avoided.
  Related article: DEXEDRINE.

Dexedrine (*Smith, Kline & French*) is a proprietary preparation of the powerful STIMULANT drug dexamphetamine sulphate, which is on the controlled drugs list. It is used primarily to treat narcolepsy (a condition marked by irresistible attacks of sleep during the daytime), although it is sometimes also used under specialist supervision to treat children who are medically hyperactive. Tolerance and dependence (addiction) are major hazards. Produced in the form of tablets, it is not generally recommended for children.

- ▲/● side-effects/warning: *see* DEXAMPHETAMINE SULPHATE.

dexfenfluramine hydrochloride is an APPETITE SUPPRESSANT drug used for the treatment of severe obesity. It is the dextro-isomer of the powerful appetite suppressant drug FENFLURAMINE. Dexfenfluramine is a sedative, rather than a stimulant as with most other appetite suppressants, and may affect a patient's thought and movement, and is potentially addictive (although dependence is rare). It is available in the form of capsules.

- ▲ side-effects: there may be depression; drowsiness, with headache, vertigo and diarrhoea and other gastrointestinal disturbances, sleep disturbances, rashes, reduction in libido. Sometimes there is insomnia, dry mouth, fluid retention, increased frequency of urination. Treatment is only in the short term, tolerance and/or dependence may occur; dosage should be tapered off gradually to avoid withdrawal depression.
- ● warning: avoid administering to patients with a history of depressive illness, drug abuse or alcoholism, epilepsy, and personality disorders, or who are pregnant or breast-feeding. Not recommended for children.
  Related article: ADIFAX.

dextromethorphan is an ANTITUSSIVE, an OPIATE that is used singly or in combination with other drugs in linctuses, syrups and lozenges to relieve dry or painful coughs.

- ▲ side-effects: constipation is a comparatively common side-effect.
- ● warning: dextromethorphan should not be administered to patients who suffer from liver disease. Used as a linctus, it may cause sputum retention which may be injurious to patients with asthma, chronic bronchitis or bronchiectasis (two conditions for which linctuses are commonly prescribed).
  Related articles: ACTIFED COMPOUND LINCTUS; COUGH

CAPS; NIGHT NURSE; TANCOLIN; VICKS COLDCARE.

dextromoramide is a synthesized derivative of morphine, and like morphine used as a NARCOTIC ANALGESIC to counter severe and intractable pain, particularly in the final stages of terminal illness. Proprietary forms are on the controlled drugs list because, also like morphine, dextromoramide is potentially addictive.

▲ side-effects: shallow breathing, urinary retention, constipation, and nausea are all common; tolerance and dependence (addiction) occur fairly readily. There may also be drowsiness, vertigo, hallucinations, effects on the cardiovascular system, and pain at the site of injection (where there may also be tissue damage).

● warning: dextromoramide should not be administered to patients who suffer from head injury, raised intracranial pressure, or who are pregnant; it should be administered with caution to those with impaired kidney or liver function, asthma, depressed respiration, insufficient secretion of thyroid hormones (hypothyroidism) or low blood pressure (hypotension), or who are lactating. Dosage should be decreased for the elderly or debilitated.

Related article: PALFIUM.

dextropropoxyphene is a weak ANALGESIC, which is nevertheless similar to a narcotic, used to treat pain anywhere in the body. It is usually combined with other analgesics (especially paracetamol or aspirin) for compound effect. Administration of the drug alone is oral in the form of capsules.

▲ side-effects: shallow breathing, urinary retention, constipation, and nausea are all common; in high overdosage tolerance and dependence (addiction) occur fairly readily, leading possibly to psychoses, convulsions and occasionally liver damage.

● warning: dextropropoxyphene should not be administered to patients who suffer from head injury or raised intracranial pressure; it should be administered with caution to those with impaired kidney or liver function, asthma, depressed respiration, insufficient secretion of thyroid hormones (hypothyroidism) or low blood pressure (hypotension), or who are pregnant or lactating. Dosage should be decreased for the elderly or debilitated. It should be avoided in porphyria.

Related articles: COSALGESIC; DISTALGESIC; DOLOXENE.

DF118 (*Duncan, Flockhart*) is a proprietary narcotic ANALGESIC available on prescription only to private patients, used to treat moderate to severe pain anywhere in the body. Produced in the form of tablets and as an elixir for dilution (the potency of the elixir once dilute is retained for 14 days) and in ampoules (as a controlled drug) for injection, DF118 is a preparation of the narcotic dihydrocodeine tartrate.

▲/● side-effects/warning: *see* DIHYDROCODEINE TARTRATE.

DHC Continus (*Napp*) is a proprietary narcotic ANALGESIC, available on prescription only, used to treat moderate to severe pain. Produced in the form of sustained-release tablets (in 3 strengths).

▲/● side-effects/warning: *see* DIHYDROCODEINE TARTRATE.

diamorphine is the chemical name of heroin, a white crystalline powder that is a

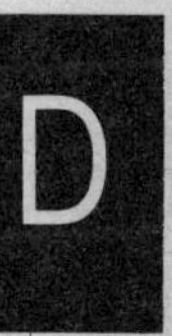

derivative of morphine. Like morphine, it is a powerful NARCOTIC ANALGESIC useful in the treatment of moderate to severe pain, although it has a shorter duration of effect; and like morphine it is also sometimes used – generally in the form of diamorphine hydrochloride – as a cough suppressant in compound linctuses (especially in the treatment of terminal lung cancer). Again like morphine, its use quickly tends to tolerance and then dependence (addiction). Administration is oral in the form of tablets or an elixir, or by injection.

▲ side-effects: there may be euphoria, depending on dosage. There may also be constipation and low blood pressure. In some patients there is respiratory depression with high dosage.

● warning: diamorphine should not be administered to patients with renal or liver disease; it should be administered with caution to those with asthma (because it tends to cause sputum retention).

Diamox (*Lederle*) is a proprietary DIURETIC, available only on prescription, used occasionally to assist in the prevention of epileptic seizures. Produced in the form of tablets, as capsules (under the trade name Diamox Sustets), and as a powder for reconstitution as a medium for injection or infusion, Diamox is a preparation of acetazolamide. It is not recommended for children.

▲/● side-effects/warning: *see* ACETAZOLAMIDE.

diazepam is an ANXIOLYTIC drug, one of the earliest of the BENZODIAZEPINES, used to treat anxiety in the short-term, to relieve insomnia, and to assist in the treatment of alcohol withdrawal symptoms and migraine. It may be used additionally to provide sedation for very minor surgery or as a premedication prior to surgical procedures and, because it also has some SKELETAL MUSCLE RELAXANT properties, to treat the spasm of tetanus or poisoning, or to relieve the bronchospasm of severe conditions of asthma. It also has an important use in the treatment of status epilepticus when given by injection. Continued use results in tolerance and may lead to dependence (addiction), especially in patients with a history of drug (including alcohol) abuse. Administration is oral in the form of tablets or capsules or a dilute elixir, topical as anal suppositories, or by injection.

▲ side-effects: there may be drowsiness, unsteadiness, headache, and shallow breathing; hypersensitivity reactions may occur.

● warning: concentration and speed of thought and movement are often affected; the effects of alcohol consumption may also be enhanced. Diazepam should be administered with caution to patients with respiratory difficulties, or kidney or liver damage; who are in the last stages of pregnancy; or who are elderly or debilitated. Prolonged use of the drug or abrupt withdrawal from treatment should be avoided.

Related articles: ATENSINE; DIAZEMULS; EVACALM; SOLIS; STESOLID; TENSIUM; VALIUM.

Diazemuls (*Dumex*) is a proprietary SEDATIVE, ANXIOLYTIC, and ANTICONVULSANT preparation of the BENZODIAZEPINE diazepam. It is produced in the form of an emulsion for injection and is intended for use in the suppression of status epilepticus,

the control of muscle spasm (e.g. in tetanus), severe agitation (e.g. with drug withdrawal symptoms), and as a sedative before surgery.
▲/✚ side-effects/warning: *see* DIAZEPAM.

diclofenac sodium is a non-steroidal, ANTI-INFLAMMATORY, non-narcotic ANALGESIC drug used to treat pain and inflammation in rheumatic disease and other musculo-skeletal disorders (such as arthritis and gout). Administration is oral in the form of tablets, topical in the form of anal suppositories, or by injection.
▲ side-effects: there may be nausea and gastrointestinal disturbance (to avoid which a patient may be advised to take the drug with food or milk), headache and ringing in the ears (tinnitus). Some patients experience sensitivity reactions (such as a rash or the symptoms of asthma). Fluid retention and/or blood disorders may occur.
✚ warning: diclofenac sodium should be administered with caution to patients with gastric ulcers, impaired kidney or liver function, or allergic disorders particularly induced by aspirin or anti-inflammatory drugs, or to those who are pregnant.
Related article: RHUMALGAN; VALENAC; VOLRAMAN; VOLTAROL.

Diconal (*Calmic*) is a proprietary NARCOTIC ANALGESIC, which is on the controlled drugs list. Used to treat moderate to severe pain, and produced in the form of tablets, Diconal represents a compound of the OPIATE dipipanone hydrochloride together with the ANTIHISTAMINE and ANTINAUSEANT cyclizine hydrochloride. It is not recommended for children or the terminally ill.
▲/✚ side-effects/warning: *see* CYCLIZINE; DIPIPANONE.

diethyl ether is the now old-fashioned 'ether' used as a general ANAESTHETIC. Powerful as it is, it is now unpopular both because it is flammable and explosive in the presence of oxygen, and because it tends to cause nausea and vomiting in a patient. All the same, it is an effective anaesthetic under the influence of which body processes – in particular the heart rhythm – are generally well maintained.

diethylpropion hydrochloride is a drug used under medical supervision to aid slimming regimes because it acts as an APPETITE SUPPRESSANT. But it is also a stimulant and potentially represents the basis for drug abuse, although the stimulant action may in fact be useful in the treatment of lethargic and/or depressed patients. Proprietary preparations are therefore on the controlled drugs list. Administration is oral in the form of sustained-release tablets.
▲ side-effects: there is rapid heart rate, nervous agitation and insomnia, tremor, gastrointestinal disturbance, dry mouth, dizziness and often headache and rashes. Tolerance and dependence may occur. Susceptible patients may undergo psychotic episodes.
✚ warning: diethylpropion hydrochloride should not be administered to patients who suffer from glaucoma or any medical condition (such as thyrotoxicosis) that disposes towards excitability, or to those suffering epilepsy or porphyria. It should also not be administered to pregnant patients or during lactation, or to those with severe hypertension or a history of drug abuse. It should be

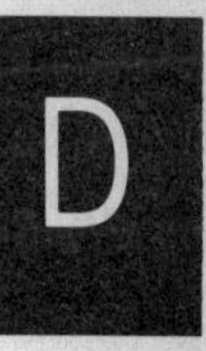

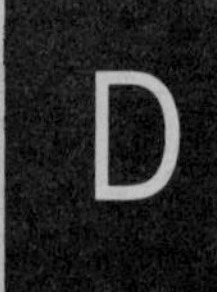

administered with caution to those with heart disease, peptic ulcer or depression. It should be avoided in children and the elderly.
Related articles: APISATE; TENUATE DOSPAN.

diflunisal is a non-steroidal, ANTI-INFLAMMATORY, non-narcotic ANALGESIC drug derived from aspirin, used to treat pain and inflammation especially in rheumatic disease and other musculo-skeletal disorders. Administration is oral in the form of tablets.
▲ side-effects: there may be nausea and gastrointestinal disturbance (to avoid which a patient may be advised to take the drug with food or milk), headache and ringing in the ears (tinnitus). Some patients experience sensitivity reactions (such as the symptoms of asthma). Fluid retention and/or blood disorders may occur.
✚ warning: diflunisal should be administered with caution to patients with gastric ulcers, impaired kidney or liver function, or allergic disorders particularly those induced by aspirin or anti-inflammatory agents, or those who are pregnant or lactating.
Related article: DOLOBID.

Dihydergot (*Sandoz*) is a proprietary preparation, available only on prescription, which is used specifically to treat migraine attacks. It also has ANTINAUSEANT properties. Produced in the form of tablets, as an oral solution, and in ampoules for injection, Dihydergot is a preparation of the ergotamine derivative dihydroergotamine mesylate
▲/✚ side-effects/warning: *see* DIHYDROERGOTAMINE MESYLATE.

dihydrocodeine tartrate is a NARCOTIC ANALGESIC that is similar to CODEINE. It is used to relieve pain, especially in cases where continued mobility is required, although it may cause some degree of dizziness and constipation. It is commonly used before and after surgery. Administration is oral in the form of tablets or a dilute elixir, or by injection.
▲ side-effects: there is dizziness, headache, and sedation; often there is also nausea and constipation. The effects of alcohol consumption may be increased.
✚ warning: dihydrocodeine tartrate should not be administered to patients with respiratory depression, obstructive airways disease, or to children aged under 12 months. Tolerance and dependence (addiction) readily occur.
Related article: DF118; DHC CONTINUS.

dihydroergotomine mesylate is an ANTIMIGRAINE drug, a derivative of ergotamine, which also has ANTINAUSEANT properties. It is used specifically to treat migraine attacks and is administered orally in the form of tablets or a solution, or by injection.
▲ side-effects: there may be nausea and vomiting, with headache, and paraesthesia, and possibly vascular spasm.
✚ warning: dihydroergotamine mesylate should not be administered to patients with any infection or circulatory disorders of the limbs, or who are pregnant or lactating; to those with heart, liver or kidney disease, or an excess of thyroid hormones in the bloodstream (thyrotoxicosis).
Related article: DIHYDERGOT.

dimenhydrinate is an ANTIHISTAMINE that is effective in quelling nausea (*see* ANTIEMETIC and ANTINAUSEANT), and useful in preventing vomiting caused by travelling in a moving vehicle, by pregnancy, or by chemotherapy or radiation sickness. It is also used to assist in the treatment of the vertigo and loss of balance that accompanies infections of the middle or inner ear. Administration is oral in the form of tablets.

▲ side-effects: there may be dry mouth, drowsiness and headache, with blurred vision. Some patients experience gastroinetstinal disturbances.

● warning: dimenhydrinate should be administered with caution to patients who suffer from liver disease, epilepsy, enlargement of the prostate gland or glaucoma, and during pregnancy. Concentration and speed of thought and movement are affected – and these symptoms may be made worse by alcohol consumption. It should be avoided in porphyria.
Related article: DRAMAMINE.

Dimotane with Codeine (*Robins*) is a proprietary, non-prescription cough linctus (ANTITUSSIVE), which is not available from the National Health Service. Intended both to promote the expulsion of excess bronchial secretions and to suppress a cough, it contains the OPIATE codeine phosphate, the ANTIHISTAMINE brompheniramine maleate and the SYMPATHOMIMETIC pseudo-ephedrine hydrochloride, and is produced as a sugar-free elixir (in two strengths, the weaker labelled for children) for dilution with glycerol (the potency of the elixir once diluted is retained for 14 days).

▲/● side-effects/warning: *see* CODEINE PHOSPHATE.

Dimyril (*Fisons*) is a proprietary cough linctus, which is available on prescription only to private patients. It represents a preparation of the ANTITUSSIVE isoaminile citrate, and is produced in the form of a syrup for dilution (the potency of the syrup once dilute is retained for 14 days).

▲/● side-effects/warning: *see* ISOAMINILE CITRATE.

diphenhydramine hydrochloride is an ANTIHISTAMINE. Its SEDATIVE properties are useful in inducing sleep in some allergic conditions, and the fact that it is also an ANTINAUSEANT makes it useful in the treatment or prevention of travel sickness, vertigo, especially due to infections of the inner and middle ears. Administration is oral in the form of capsules.

▲ side-effects: sedation may affect patients' capacity for speed of thought and movement; there may be headache and/or weight gain, dry mouth, gastrointestinal disturbances and visual problems.

● warning: diphenhydramine hydrochloride should not be administered to patients with glaucoma, urinary retention, intestinal obstruction, enlargement of the prostate gland, or peptic ulcer, or who are pregnant; it should be administered with caution to those who suffer from epilepsy or liver disease.
Related articles: BENADRYL; HISTALIX.

dipipanone is a rapidly-acting and powerful OPIATE, NARCOTIC, ANALGESIC drug, which is used in combination with an

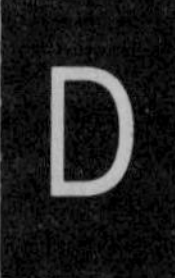

ANTINAUSEANT drug (the ANTIHISTAMINE cyclizine) for the relief of acute moderate to severe pain. Its proprietary form is on the controlled drugs list and is not recommended for children. Administration (in the form of dipipanone hydrochloride) is oral as tablets.

▲ side-effects: the mouth may become dry, vision may blur, and the patient may become drowsy. Hallucinations, mood changes, palpitations, difficulties in urination, bradycardia (low heart rate) may also be experienced. Tolerance may rapidly be followed by dependence (addiction).

✚ warning: dipipanone should not be administered to patients who have any blockage of the respiratory passages or any form of depressed breathing, or to those with raised intracranial pressure or head injuries; it should be administered with caution to those with severely impaired kidney or liver function, or who are pregnant. The consumption of alcohol must be avoided during treatment. *Related article:* DICONAL.

dipotassium clorazepate is a drug better known simply as clorazepate, used for short-term anxiety.
see CLORAZEPATE.

Diprivan (*ICI*) is a proprietary form of the general ANAESTHETIC propofol, used primarily for the induction of anaesthesia at the start of a surgical operation, but sometimes also for its maintenance thereafter. Available only in hospital, it is produced as an emulsion in ampoules for injection.
▲/✚ side-effects/warning: *see* PROPOFOL.

Disalcid (*Riker*) is a proprietary, ANTI-INFLAMMATORY non-narcotic ANALGESIC, available only on prescription, used to relieve pain – particularly the pain of rheumatic disease in and around the joints. Produced in the form of tablets, it represents a preparation of the aspirin-like drug salsalate, and is not recommended for children.
▲/✚ side-effects/warning: *see* SALSALATE.

Disipal (*Brocades*) is a proprietary ANTICHOLINERGIC drug, available only on prescription, used in ANTIPARKINSONIAN treatment to relieve some of the symptoms of parkinsonism, specifically the tremor of the hands, the overall rigidity of the posture, and the tendency to produce an excess of saliva. (The drug also has the capacity to treat these conditions in some cases where they are produced by drugs.) It is thought to work by compensating for the lack of the neurotransmitter DOPAMINE in the brain that is the major cause of such parkinsonian symptoms. Produced in the form of tablets, Disipal is a preparation of orphenadrine hydrochloride. Counselling of patients is advised.
▲/✚ side-effects/warning: *see* ORPHENADRINE HYDROCHLORIDE.

Disprin (*Reckitt & Colman*) is a proprietary, non-prescription, non-narcotic ANALGESIC containing paracetomol.
▲/✚ side-effects/warning: *see* PARACETAMOL.

Disprol (*Reckitt & Colman*) is a proprietary, non-prescription, non-narcotic ANALGESIC for children which also helps to reduce high body temperature. Produced in the form of a sugar-free suspension, it is a preparation of paracetamol. Even as a paediatric preparation,

however, it is not recommended for children aged under 3 months.
▲/◆ side-effects/warning: *see* PARACETAMOL.

Distalgesic (*Dista*) is a proprietary ANALGESIC available only on prescription to private patients. Used to relieve pain anywhere in the body, and produced in the form of tablets, Distalgesic is a preparation of the narcotic-like analgesic dextropropoxyphene together with paracetamol. This compound combination is known as CO-PROXAMOL). It is not recommended for children.
▲/◆ side-effects/warning: *see* DEXTROPROPOXYPHENE; PARACETAMOL.

disulfiram is a drug used as an adjunct in the treatment of alcoholism. In combination with the consumption of even small quantities of alcohol, it gives rise to unpleasant, even dangerous, reactions – such as flushing, headache, palpitations, nausea and vomiting. This is because disulfiram and alcohol together cause an accumulation in the body of acetaldehyde, which is toxic. The drug is quite well known under its proprietary name Antabuse. Administration is oral in the form of tablets.
▲ side-effects: taken with a large amount of alcohol the drug may cause low blood pressure, serious heartbeat irregularities, and eventual collapse.
◆ warning: disulfiram should not be administered to patients with certain heart disorders, or during pregnancy, or to patients with drug dependence or mental illness. Simultaneous use of medications containing forms of alcohol should be carefully avoided.
Related article: ANTABUSE.

Dixarit (*WB Pharmaceuticals*) is a proprietary preparation of the drug clonidine hydrochloride, used in low dosage sometimes as an ANTIMIGRAINE drug to try to prevent recurrent migraine and similar headaches. It is produced in the form of tablets, and is not recommended for children.
▲/◆ side-effects/warning: *see* CLONIDINE HYDROCHLORIDE.

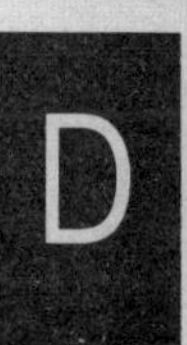

Dolmatil (*Squibb*) is a proprietary ANTIPSYCHOTIC drug used to treat the symptoms of schizophrenia. In low doses it increases an apathetic, withdrawn patient's awareness and tends to generate a true consciousness of events. In high doses it is used also to treat other conditions that may cause tremor, tics, involuntary movements or involuntary utterances (such as the relatively uncommon Giles de la Tourette syndrome). Produced in the form of tablets, Dolmatil is a preparation of sulpiride. It is not recommended for children aged under 14 years.
▲/◆ side-effects/warning: *see* SULPIRIDE.

Dolobid (*Morson*) is a proprietary, ANTI-INFLAMMATORY, non-narcotic ANALGESIC, available only on prescription, used to treat the pain of rheumatic disease and other musculo-skeletal disorders. Produced in the form of tablets (in two strengths), Dolobid is a preparation of the aspirin-like, anti-inflammatory drug diflunisal. It is not recommended for children.
▲/◆ side-effects/warning: *see* DIFLUNISAL.

Doloxene (*Lilly*) is a proprietary, narcotic ANALGESIC, available on prescription only to private patients, used to treat mild to moderate pain anywhere in the body. Produced in the form of capsules, Doloxene is a

preparation of the OPIATE-like dextropropoxyphene napsylate. It is not recommended for children.
▲/ ⬣ side-effects/warning: *see* DEXTROPROPOXYPHENE.

D

Domical (*Berk*) is a proprietary ANTIDEPRESSANT drug, available only on prescription, administered to treat depressive illness (and especially in cases where some degree of sedation is deemed necessary). Like many such drugs, it is also used to treat bedwetting by children at night. Produced in the form of tablets (in three strengths), Domical is a preparation of the tricyclic antidepressant amitriptyline.
▲/ ⬣ side-effects/warning: *see* AMITRIPTYLINE.

domperidone is an ANTI-EMETIC drug that is thought to work by inhibiting the action of the neurotransmitter DOPAMINE in the brain; this can be useful in patients undergoing treatment with cytotoxic drugs. It is also used to prevent vomiting in patients treated for parkinsonism with levodopa or bromocriptine. Administration is oral in the form of tablets or in suspension, or as anal suppositories.
▲ side-effects: occasionally, spontaneous lactation in women or the development of feminine breasts in men may occur.
⬣ warning: domperidone should be administered with caution to those who suffer from impaired kidney function, who are pregnant or lactating. Prolonged treatment is not desirable.
Related article: MOTILIUM.

dopamine is a NEUROTRANSMITTER substance (a catecholamine), in its own right, in the brain. It is also an intermediate in the synthesis of another important neurotransmitter NORADRENALINE. It is possible that some psychoses may in part be caused by abnormalities in the release, activity and metabolism of dopamine in the brain, because drugs that antagonize its activity as a neurotransmitter (such as chlorpromazine) tend to relieve some of the more positive and disturbing symptoms of schizophrenia. Drugs mimicking some of the actions of dopamine may be beneficial in the treatment of some cases of Parkinson's Disease, where there is a gradual loss of nerves containing this neurotransmitter. The drug LEVODOPA works in this treatment by conversion to dopamine within the brain.

Dopram (*Robins*) is a proprietary preparation of the respiratory stimulant drug doxapram hydrochloride, available only on prescription, used in some instances to relieve severe respiratory difficulties in patients with chronic disease of the respiratory tract or who undergo respiratory depression following major surgery, particularly in cases where ventilatory support is for one reason or another not applicable. It is produced in flasks (bottles) for infusion (in dextrose solution) or in ampoules for injection.
▲/ ⬣ side-effects/warning: *see* DOXAPRAM HYDROCHLORIDE.

Dormonoct (*Roussel*) is a proprietary HYPNOTIC drug, available only on prescription, used in the short term to treat insomnia. Produced in the form of tablets, it is a preparation of the BENZODIAZEPINE loprazolam mesylate. It is not recommended for children.
▲/ ⬣ side-effects/warning: *see* LOPRAZOLAM.

dothiepin hydrochloride is a TRICYCLIC ANTIDEPRESSANT drug used to treat depressive illness, especially in cases where some degree of sedation is deemed to be necessary. Administration is oral in the form of capsules or tablets.

▲ side-effects: common effects include sedation (affecting driving ability), dry mouth and blurred vision; there may also be difficulty in urinating, sweating and irregular heartbeat, behavioural disturbances, a rash, a state of confusion, and/or a loss of libido. Rarely, there are also blood disorders.

● warning: dothiepin hydrochloride should not be administered to patients who suffer from heart disease or psychosis; it should be administered with caution to patients who suffer from diabetes, epilepsy, liver or thyroid disease, glaucoma or urinary retention; or who are pregnant or lactating. Withdrawal of treatment must be gradual.
Related article: PROTHIADEN.

doxapram hydrochloride is a respiratory stimulant drug, used with care in some instances, to relieve severe respiratory difficulties in patients who suffer from chronic disease of the respiratory tract or who undergo respiratory depression following major surgery, particularly in cases where ventilatory support is not applicable. Administration is by injection or by infusion (in dextrose solution).

▲ side-effects: the blood pressure and heart rate may increase; some patients experience dizziness.

● warning: doxapram hydrochloride should not be administered to patients who suffer from very high blood pressure (hypertension), from cardiovascular disease, from an excess of thyroid hormones in the blood (thyrotoxicosis), or from severe asthma; it should be administered with caution to those who suffer from epilepsy or who are taking antidepressant drugs that affect mood.
Related article: DOPRAM.

doxepin is a TRICYCLIC ANTIDEPRESSANT drug used to treat depressive illness, especially in cases where some degree of sedation is deemed to be necessary. Administration is oral in the form of capsules (comprising doxepin hydrochloride).

▲ side-effects: common effects include sedation (affecting driving ability), dry mouth and blurred vision; there may also be difficulty in urinating, sweating and irregular heartbeat, behavioural disturbances, a rash, a state of confusion, and/or a loss of libido. Rarely, there are also blood disorders.

● warning: doxepin should not be administered to patients who suffer from heart disease or psychosis; it should be administered with caution to patients who suffer from diabetes, epilepsy, liver or thyroid disease, glaucoma or urinary retention; or who are pregnant. It should be avoided in lactating women. Withdrawal of treatment must be gradual.
Related article: SINEQUAN.

Dozic (*RP Drugs*) is a proprietary ANTIPSYCHOTIC drug, available only on prescription, used to treat psychosis (especially schizophrenia or the centrally hyperactive condition mania) and to tranquillize patients undergoing behavioural disturbance. It may also be used in the short term to treat severe anxiety. Produced in the form of a sugar-free liquid (for swallowing, in two strengths), Dozic is a

preparation of the drug haloperidol.
▲/✚ side-effects/warning: *see* HALOPERIDOL.

Dramamine (*Searle*) is a proprietary, non-prescription ANTI-EMETIC, used to treat nausea and vomiting, to prevent forms of motion sickness, and to relieve the loss of balance and vertigo experienced by patients with infections of the middle or inner ear or who have radiation sickness. Produced in the form of tablets, Dramamine is a preparation of dimenhydrinate. It is not recommended for children aged under 12 months.
▲/✚ side-effects/warning: *see* DIMENHYDRINATE.

Droleptan (*Janssen*) is a proprietary preparation of the powerful major TRANQUILLIZER droperidol, available only on prescription, used primarily in emergencies to subdue or soothe psychotic (particularly manic) patients during behavioural disturbances, although it is also used on patients about to undergo certain diagnostic procedures that may be difficult or painful, because it promotes a sensation of dispassionate detachment. It is produced in the form of tablets, as a sugar-free liquid for dilution (the potency of the liquid once dilute is retained for 14 days), and in ampoules for injection.
▲/✚ side-effects/warning: *see* DROPERIDOL.

droperidol is a major TRANQUILLIZER and ANTIPSYCHOTIC of the butyrophenone class, used primarily in emergencies to subdue or soothe psychotic (particularly manic) patients during behavioural disturbances, although it is also used on patients about to undergo certain diagnostic procedures that may be difficult or painful, because it promotes a sensation of dispassionate detachment. It is used as an ANTI-EMETIC for nausea and vomiting caused by chemotherapy, and as an adjunct to general anaesthetics for surgery. Administration is oral in the form of tablets or as a sugar-free dilute liquid, or by injection.
▲ side-effects: concentration and speed of reaction is usually affected. There may also be restlessness, insomnia and nightmares, rashes and jaundice, dry mouth, gastrointestinal disturbances, difficulties in urinating, and blurred vision. Extrapyramidal motor side-effects may occur, e.g. muscles in the neck and back, and sometimes in the arms, may undergo spasms. Rarely, there is weight loss and impaired kidney function.
✚ warning: droperidol should not be administered to patients with a reduction in the bone-marrow's capacity to produce blood cells, or with certain types of glaucoma. It should be administered only with caution to those with heart or vascular disease, kidney or liver disease, parkinsonism, or depression; or who are pregnant or lactating.
Related articles: DROLEPTAN; THALAMONAL.

Duromine (*Riker*) is a proprietary preparation of phentermine, which, as a strong STIMULANT drug, is on the controlled drugs list. Used as an APPETITE SUPPRESSANT in the medical treatment of obesity, it is produced in the form of sustained-release tablets (in two strengths), and is not recommended for children.
▲/✚ side-effects/warning: *see* PHENTERMINE.

Ebufac (*DDSA Pharmaceuticals*) is a proprietary, non-narcotic ANALGESIC that has additional ANTI-INFLAMMATORY properties. Available only on prescription, Ebufac is used to relieve pain – particularly the pain of rheumatic disease and other musculo-skeletal disorders – and is produced in the form of tablets consisting of a preparation of ibuprofen.
▲/✚ side-effects/warning: *see* IBUPROFEN.

Effico (*Pharmax*) is a proprietary, non-prescription tonic, which is not available from the National Health Service. Used primarily as an appetite stimulant, Effico contains the STIMULANT caffeine, vitamin B in the form of thiamine hydrochloride and nicotinamide, and an infusion of gentian. It is produced in the form of a syrup for dilution (the potency of the syrup once dilute is retained for 14 days).
▲/✚ side-effects/warning: *see* CAFFEINE.

Efufac (*Cox, DDSA*) is a proprietary form of the non-steroidal, ANTI-INFLAMMATORY (NSAID), non-narcotic, ANALAGESIC drug ibuprofen. Available on prescription, it is used to treat pain and inflammation particularly that caused by musculo-skeletal disorders. Administrationis in the form of tablets (in three strengths).
▲/✚ side-effects/warning: *see* IBUPROFEN.

Elavil (*DDSA Pharmaceuticals*) is a proprietary ANTIDEPRESSANT drug, available only on prescription, administered to treat depressive illness (and especially in cases where some degree of sedation is deemed necessary). Like many such drugs, it has also been used to treat bedwetting by children at night although this use is now becoming less common. Produced in the form of tablets (in two strengths), Elavil is a preparation of the TRICYCLIC ANTIDEPRESSANT amitriptyline hydrochloride.
▲/✚ side-effects/warning: *see* AMITRIPTYLINE.

Emeside (*L A B*) is a proprietary preparation of the ANTI-EPILEPTIC drug ethosuximide, available only on prescription, used to treat and suppress petit mal ('absence') seizures. Produced in the form of capsules and as a blackcurrant- or orange-flavoured syrup for dilution (the potency of the syrup once diluted is retained for 14 days), Emeside's effects should be monitored following the initiation of treatment so that an optimum treatment level can be established.
▲/✚ side-effects/warning: *see* ETHOSUXIMIDE.

***emetic** is any agent that causes vomiting. Emetics are used mostly to treat poisoning by non-acidic, non-corrosive substances, especially drugs in overdose. Some affect the vomiting centre in the brain; others irritate the stomach nerves. *see* ANTI-EMETIC.

enflurane is a volatile general ANAESTHETIC usually given to supplement nitrous oxide-oxygen mixtures (in a concentration of between 1 and 5%) for the induction and maintenance of anaesthesia during major surgery. Only a small proportion of the drug is metabolized by a patient, making it particularly safe for repeated use. Administration is by inhalation through a calibrated vaporizer.
▲ side-effects: reduced heart function results in low blood pressure.
✚ warning: enflurane slows both the heart and the breathing rate. Shallow breathing may

E

tend to build up carbon dioxide levels in the body. The drug should not be administered to patients who have respiratory disorders.
Related article: ETHRANE.

Enflurane (*Abbott*) is a proprietary form of the volatile general ANAESTHETIC enflurane.
▲/ ● side-effects/warning: *see* ENFLURANE.

***enzymes** are substances within the body that play an essential part in metabolism since they act as catalysts in speeding the rate of specific necessary biochemical reactions. Some drugs exert their actions through inhibiting or increasing the activity of these natural components of the body, and in rarer instances enzymes are administered to patients in which case they are regarded as drugs since these chemicals are now foreign to the body. Examples of the former are the ANTIDEPRESSANT drugs MAO INHIBITORS, and of the latter cristanaspase.

Epanutin (*Parke-Davis*) is a proprietary ANTICONVULSANT drug, available only on prescription, used to treat and prevent grand mal (tonic-clonic) and partial (focal) epileptic seizures. It is sometimes alternatively used to treat trigeminal (facial) neuralgia. Produced in the form of capsules (in three strengths), as chewable tablets (under the name Epanutin Infatabs), and as a suspension for dilution (the potency of the suspension once dilute is retained for 14 days), Epanutin is a preparation of the drug phenytoin.
▲/ ● side-effects/warning: *see* PHENYTOIN.

Epanutin Ready Mixed Parenteral (*Parke-Davis*) is a form of the proprietary ANTICONVULSANT drug EPANUTIN, which is administered to treat the emergency epileptic condition status epilepticus. It may, however, also be used to prevent convulsive seizures during neurosurgical operations and, also to treat and regularize heartbeat irregularities. Produced in ampoules for injection, it is a solution of phenytoin sodium with propylene glycol. Not recommended for children.
▲/ ● side-effects/warning: *see* PHENYTOIN.

Epilim (*Labaz*) is a proprietary ANTICONVULSANT drug, available only on prescription, used to treat all forms of epilepsy. Considerable monitoring of body functions is necessary during treatment for the first 6 months. Produced in the form of crushable tablets, as enteric-coated tablets (in two strengths), as a sugar-free liquid, as a syrup for dilution (the potency of the syrup once dilute is retained for 14 days), and as a powder for reconstitution as a solution for injection, Epilim Intravenous. Epilim is a preparation of the carboxylic acid derivative sodium valproate.
▲/ ● side-effects/warning: *see* SODIUM VALPROATE.

Equagesic (*Wyeth*) is a proprietary compound ANALGESIC, which is on the controlled drugs list and is not available from the National Health Service. Used primarily in the short-term treatment of rheumatic pain or the symptoms of other musculo-skeletal disorders, and produced in the form of tablets, Equagesic contains the (potentially addictive) TRANQUILLIZER meprobamate, the SKELETAL MUSCLE RELAXANT ethoheptazine citrate, and the non-narcotic analgesic aspirin. It is not recommended for children. There

are interactions with a wide variety of drugs including alcohol and nervous system depressants.
▲/● side-effects/warning: *see* ASPIRIN; MEPROBAMATE.

Equanil (*Wyeth*) is a proprietary ANXIOLYTIC drug that is on the controlled drugs list. Used in the short-term treatment of nervous anxiety and associated muscular tension, and produced in the form of tablets (in two strengths), Equanil is a preparation of the, potentially addictive, TRANQUILLIZER meprobamate. It is not recommended for children, and is contraindicated in acute porphyria and alcoholism.
▲/● side-effects/warning: *see* MEPROBAMATE.

ergotamine tartrate is an ANTIMIGRAINE drug administered to patients who suffer from migraine, which is not relieved by analgesics. A vegetable alkaloid, it is most effectively administered during the aura – the initial symptoms – of an attack, and probably works by constricting the cranial arteries. However, although the pain may be relieved, other symptoms, such as the visual disturbances and nausea, may not (although other drugs may be administered to treat those separately). Repeated treatment may in some patients eventually lead to habituation (addiction); in others it may cause ergot poisoning, resulting in gangrene of the fingers and toes, and confusion. Administration is oral in the form of tablets either for swallowing or to be held under the tongue to dissolve, or as an aerosol inhalant; one proprietary compound preparation is in the form of anal suppositories.
▲ side-effects: there may be abdominal pain and muscle cramps that may lead to nausea and vomiting. Overdosage or rapid withdrawal of the drug may in turn cause headache.
● warning: ergotamine tartrate should not be administered to patients who suffer from vascular disease or any infection, or who are pregnant or lactating. It should be administered with caution to those with kidney, liver or heart disease, or with thyroid gland overactivity. Dosage should be carefully monitored; treatment should not be repeated within 4 days. It should never be administered on a prophylactic (preventative) basis. Treatment should be withdrawn at once if the patient experiences tingling or numbness at the extremities.
Related articles: CAFERGOT; LINGRAINE; MEDIHALER-ERGOTAMINE; MIGRIL.

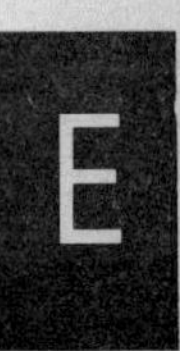

ethamivan is a respiratory stimulant drug, used occasionally to relieve severe respiratory difficulties in patients who suffer from chronic disease of the respiratory tract, or who undergo respiratory depression following major surgery – especially in cases where for one reason or another ventilatory support is not applicable. Administration is oral in the form of a solution or by injection.
▲ side-effects: there may be nausea, restlessness and tremor, leading possibly to convulsions and heartbeat irregularities.
● warning: ethamivan should not be administered to patients who have respiratory failure due to drug overdose or neurological disease, or with coronary artery disease, severe asthma, or an excess of thyroid hormones in the blood (thyrotoxicosis). It should be administered with caution to those with severe high blood pressure (hypertension) or a

reduced supply of blood to the heart. It should not be administered to children. *Related article:* CLAIRVAN.

E

ethanol, or ethyl alcohol, is the form of alcohol found in alcoholic drinks, produced by the fermentation of sugar by yeast. *see* ALCOHOL.

ethosuximide is an ANTICONVULSANT drug used to treat and suppress a form of epilepsy found in children called petit mal ('absence') seizures. It may be used singly or in combination with other drugs, and is particularly useful in successfully treating some patients on whom other anticonvulsants have no effect. Dosage must be adjusted to the optimum level for each individual patient.
Administration is oral in the form of capsules or as a dilute elixir.
▲ side-effects: there may be gastrointestinal disturbances, drowsiness, headache and/or dizziness; some patients experience depression or euphoria. Rarely, there are haematological disorders or psychotic states.
✱ warning: ethosuximide should not be administered to patients with porphyria. Withdrawal of treatment, if undertaken, must be gradual. Special monitoring of blood levels of the drug are required for a patient who is pregnant or lactating. *Related articles:* EMESIDE, ZARONTIN.

Ethrane (*Abbott*) is a proprietary preparation of the general ANAESTHETIC enflurane, usually administered to supplement nitrous oxide-oxygen mixtures for the induction and maintenance of anaesthesia during major surgery. It is produced in gas bottles for administration through a calibrated vaporizer.
▲/✱ side-effects/warning: *see* ENFLURANE.

ethyl alcohol, or ETHANOL, is the form of alcohol found in alcoholic drinks, produced by the fermentation of carbohydrates by yeast.
see ALCOHOL.

etodolac is a non-steroidal, ANTI-INFLAMMATORY, non-narcotic ANALGESIC used primarily to treat rheumatoid arthritis.
Administration is oral in the form of tablets and capsules.
▲ side-effects: there may be gastrointestinal disturbance (which may be decreased by taking the drug with food). Some patients experience sensitivity reactions, such as a rash, and CNS side-effects, including headaches, vertigo or hearing disturbances. There may be fluid retention and consequent weight gain. Blood disorders have occurred.
✱ warning: etodolac should not be administered to patients known to be allergic to aspirin, who suffer from peptic ulcer or from gastrointestinal bleeding, or who are pregnant or lactating. It should be administered with caution to those who suffer from impaired kidney or liver function. *Related article:* LODINE.

etomidate is a general ANAESTHETIC used specifically for the initial induction of anaesthesia. Recovery after treatment is rapid and without any hangover effect, and it causes less of a fall in blood pressure than many other anaesthetics. But there is pain on injection, when there may also be simultaneous extraneous muscle movements.
▲ side-effects: repeated doses may suppress the secretion of corticosteroid hormones by the adrenal glands.

warning: pain on injection may be overcome by prior administration of suitable premedication (such as a narcotic analgesic). Intravenous injection must be carried out with caution in order to avoid thrombophlebitis.
Related article: HYPNOMIDATE.

Evacalm (*Unimed*) is a proprietary ANXIOLYTIC drug, available on prescription only to private patients, used to treat anxiety and insomnia, or to assist in the treatment of acute alcohol withdrawal symptoms. Produced in the form of tablets (in two strengths), Evacalm is a preparation of the long-acting BENZODIAZEPINE diazepam.
▲/ ✚ side-effects/warning: *see* DIAZEPAM.

Evadyne (*Ayerst*) is a proprietary, TRICYCLIC ANTIDEPRESSANT drug, available only on prescription, used to treat depression with the added complication of anxiety. Produced in the form of tablets (in two strengths), Evadyne is a preparation of butriptyline. It is not recommended for children.
▲/ ✚ side-effects/warning: *see* BUTRIPTYLINE.

Expulin (*Galen*) is a proprietary, non-prescription cough linctus (ANTITUSSIVE) that is not available from the National Health Service. It is produced as a linctus in two strengths (the weaker labelled as a paediatric version) for dilution (the potency of the linctus once dilute is retained for 14 days), and is a combination of the OPIATE pholcodine, the SYMPATHOMIMETIC ephedrine hydrochloride, the ANTIHISTAMINE chlorpheniramine maleate, and glycerol and menthol. Even the paediatric linctus is not recommended for children aged under 3 months.
▲/ ✚ side-effects/warning: *see* PHOLCODINE.

E

F

Faverin (*Duphar*) is a proprietary form of the ANTIDEPRESSANT drug fluvoxamine maleate, which has less sedative effects than some drugs of this type. Available only on prescription, as tablets in two strengths.

▲/✚ side-effects/warning: *see* FLUVOXAMINE MALEATE.

Feldene (*Pfizer*) is a proprietary, non-steroidal ANTI-INFLAMMATORY, ANALGESIC drug available only on prescription, used to treat gout, arthritic and rheumatic pain, and other musculo-skeletal disorders. Produced in the form of capsules (in two strengths), soluble (dispersible) tablets (in two strengths), as a gel, and as anal suppositories, Feldene's active constituent is piroxicam. It is not recommended for children.

▲/✚ side-effects/warning: *see* PIROXICAM.

Fenbid (*Smith, Kline & French*) is a proprietary, ANTI-INFLAMMATORY, non-narcotic ANALGESIC, available only on prescription, used to treat pain of all kinds, especially pain from arthritis and rheumatism, and other musculo-skeletal disorders. Produced in the form of spansules (sustained-release capsules), Fenbid's active constituent is ibuprofen. It is not recommended for children or patients suffering from peptic ulcer.

▲/✚ side-effects/warning: *see* IBUPROFEN.

fenbufen is an ANTI-INFLAMMATORY, non-narcotic ANALGESIC drug with effects similar to those of aspirin. It is used particularly in the treatment of pain from rheumatoid arthritis and osteoarthritis.

▲ side-effects: there may be a skin rash (the drug should then be discontinued); rarely, there is an allergic response, headache, disturbance of the sense of balance, gastrointestinal bleeding (though less than with some others of this class) or kidney dysfunction.

✚ warning: fenbufen should not be administered to patients who are pregnant or lactating; who are allergic to aspirin or other anti-inflammatory drugs; or who are already taking aspirin or an anticoagulant.
Related article: LEDERFEN.

fenfluramine hydrochloride is a drug used to aid slimming regimes because it acts as an APPETITE SUPPRESSANT. Not a stimulant – unlike most other appetite suppressants – fenfluramine hydrochloride instead has SEDATIVE properties that may affect a patient's intricacy of thought and movement, and is potentially addictive (although dependence is rare).

▲ side-effects: there may be depression; sedation, with headache, vertigo and gastric upsets, is not uncommon. Sometimes there is insomnia, dry mouth, fluid retention, increased frequency of urination and speeding of the heart rate. Treatment is only in the short term, tolerance and/or dependence may occur; dosage should be tapered off gradually to avoid withdrawal depression.

✚ warning: fenfluramine hydrochloride may affect mental concentration; it may enhance the effect of alcohol.
Related articles: ADIFAX; PONDERAX.

fenoprofen is an ANTI-INFLAMMATORY, non-narcotic ANALGESIC drug with effects similar to those of aspirin. It is used particularly in the treatment of pain from rheumatoid arthritis and osteoarthritis, and to reduce fever.

▲ side-effects: there may be a skin rash; rarely, there is an allergic response or gastrointestinal bleeding.

✚ warning: fenoprofen should not be administered to patients who are suffering from gastric or intestinal bleeding (as with a peptic ulcer); who are pregnant or lactating; who are allergic to aspirin or other anti-inflammatory drugs; who have reduced kidney function; who are asthmatic; or who are already taking aspirin, an anticoagulant or a drug to control the blood level of glucose.

Related articles: FENOPRON; PROGESIC.

Fenopron (*Dista*) is a proprietary, ANTI-INFLAMMATORY, non-narcotic ANALGESIC drug available only on prescription, used to relieve pain – particularly arthritic and rheumatic pain – and to treat other musculo-skeletal disorders. Its active constituent is fenoprofen, and it is produced in the form of tablets (in either of two strengths). It is not recommended for children.

▲/✚ side-effects/warning: *see* FENOPROFEN.

fentanyl is a NARCOTIC ANALGESIC, used primarily for analgesia during surgery and to supplement other anaesthetics; it may be used also to slow the breathing of an anaesthetized patient. As a narcotic, its proprietary forms are on the controlled drugs list.

▲ side-effects: post-operatively there may be respiratory depression, low blood pressure, slowing of the heart, and nausea (with or without vomiting).

✚ warning: fentanyl should not be administered to patients whose respiration is already impaired by disease or those with myasthenia gravis, hypothyroidism or chronic liver disease. Administration to a mother during childbirth may cause respiratory depression in the newborn. Elderly patients should be given a reduced dosage.

Related articles: SUBLIMAZE; THALAMONAL.

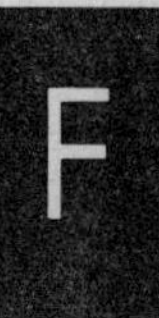

Fentazin (*Allen & Hanburys*) is a proprietary ANTIPSYCHOTIC drug, available only on prescription, used to treat and tranquillize patients who are undergoing behavioural disturbances, or who are psychotic, particularly schizophrenic. It is also used to treat severe anxiety, or as an ANTI-EMETIC and SEDATIVE prior to surgery. Produced in the form of tablets (in three strengths), Fentazin is a preparation of perphenazine. It is not recommended for children.

▲/✚ side-effects/warning: *see* PERPHENAZINE.

Flexis Continus (*Napp*) is a proprietary form of the non-steroidal, ANTI-INFLAMMATORY, non-narcotic ANALGESIC drug indomethacin. It is available on prescription as sustained-release tablets to treat pain and inflammation associated with musculo-skeletal disorders, such as rheumatic disease.

▲/✚ side-effects/warning: *see* INDOMETHACIN.

Fluanxol (*Lundbeck*) is an atypical proprietary ANTIDEPRESSANT and ANTIPSYCHOTIC, available only on prescription, used to treat depressive illness. Produced in the form of tablets (in two strengths), it represents a preparation of the primary antipsychotic compound flupenthixol, and is not

recommended for children.
▲/● side-effects/warning: *see* FLUPENTHIXOL.

flumazenil is a BENZODIAZEPINE antagonist used to reverse the central sedative effects of benzodiazepines in anaesthesia, intensive care and diagnostic procedures. Administration is by slow intravenous infusion or injection.
▲ side-effects: nausea, vomiting and flushing; agitation, anxiety and fear if wakening is too rapid, occasionally convulsions. With intensive-care patients, transient increase in blood pressure and heart rate.
● warning: flumazenil should be given with caution to high-risk or anxious patients and following major surgery, and to those with impaired liver function. It should not be administered to epileptics who have received prolonged benzodiazepine therapy.
Related article: ANEXATE

F

flunitrazepam is a BENZODIAZEPINE drug used as a HYPNOTIC to treat, in the short-term only, insomnia cases where some degree of sedation during the daytime is acceptable. Doses may have residual effects that make the overall treatment cumulative. Administration is oral, in the form of tablets.
▲ side-effects: there may be drowsiness and dry mouth. Hypersensitivity reactions sometimes occur. Prolonged use may result in tolerance and eventual dependence (addiction).
● warning: there may be a hangover following prolonged use; abrupt withdrawal is thus to be avoided. Patients should not drink alcohol. Dosage should be reduced for the elderly and the debilitated. Flunitrazepam should be administered with caution to patients who have kidney or liver damage; or who are pregnant or lactating.
Related article: ROHYPNOL.

Fluothane (*ICI*) is a proprietary form of the volatile general ANAESTHETIC halothane.
▲/● side-effects/warning: *see* HALOTHANE.

fluoxetine hydrochloride is an ANTIDEPRESSANT drug used to treat depressive illness. It has the advantage over some other antidepressant drugs that it works by inhibiting uptake of the neurotransmitter SEROTONIN, and so has relatively less SEDATIVE and ANTICHOLINERGIC side-effects. It is used as tablets.
▲ side-effects: it may impair performance of skilled tasks such as driving; may cause a rash (if so discontinue treatment), convulsions, fever, headache, tremor, nausea, vomiting, diarrhoea (which may be severe), anorexia with weight loss, slowing of the heart, hypothermia, sexual dysfunction; and occasionally blood disorders, vaginal bleeding on withdrawal, and confusion.
● warning: it should be given with caution to patients with liver or kidney damage, and those who have epilepsy, diabetes mellitus, or who are pregnant. It should be avoided in lactating women. MAO inhibitors should not be used until at least five weeks after discontinuing fluoxetine hydrochloride.
Related article: PROZAC.

flupenthixol is an ANTIPSYCHOTIC drug of the thioxanthene class used to treat psychoses, such as in schizophrenia. Because it is less sedative than many antipsychotics it may be useful in the more withdrawn subject. It has also been of value in the treatment of some depressed patients.

▲ side-effects: extrapyramidal motor disturbances (dystonias, tremor, rigidity, akathisia) are fairly common and tardive dyskinesias may occur with prolonged use. Insomina may also occur as well as hormonal disorders.

● warning: flupenthixol should not be administered to patients suffering porphyrias, who are excitable or overactive, and should be administered only with extreme caution to patients who suffer from heart, vascular, kidney, or liver disease, or parkinsonism, and who are pregnant or lactating. Dosage should be reduced for the elderly; it is not suitable for children.

Related articles: DEPIXOL; FLUANXOL.

fluphenazine is an ANTIPSYCHOTIC drug of the phenothiazine class. It is used for the treatment of psychoses, such as in schizophrenia, or the short-term control of severe manic, violent or agitated states. In its hydrochloride form it can be taken orally, but for patients who are not reliable in taking tablets it is available, as the deconoate, for depot intramuscular injection.

▲ side-effects: extrapyramidal motor disturbances (dystonias, tremor, rigidity, akathisia) are fairly common and tardive dyskinesias may occur with prolonged use. Insomina may also occur as well as hormonal disorders.

● warning: fluphenazine should be administered only with extreme caution to patients who suffer from heart or vascular disease, from kidney or liver disease, from parkinsonism, or from depression; or who are pregnant or lactating. Dosage should be reduced for the elderly; it is not suitable for children.

Related articles: MODECATE; MODITEN.

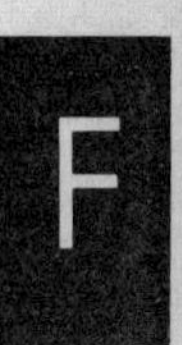

flurazepam is a BENZODIAZEPINE drug used as a HYPNOTIC to treat insomnia in cases where some degree of sedation during the daytime is acceptable. Doses may have residual effects that make the overall treatment cumulative. Administration is oral, in the form of capsules.

▲ side-effects: there may be drowsiness and dry mouth. Hypersensitivity reactions sometimes occur. Prolonged use may result in tolerance and eventual dependence (addiction).

● warning: there may be a hangover following prolonged use; abrupt withdrawal is thus to be avoided. Patients should not drink alcohol. Dosage should be reduced for the elderly and the debilitated. Flurazepam should be administered with caution to patients who have kidney or liver damage; or who are pregnant or lactating; or who have obstructive lung disease or respiratory depression.

Related article: DALMANE.

flurbiprofen is a non-steroidal ANTI-INFLAMMATORY non-narcotic ANALGESIC with effects similar to those of aspirin. It is used particularly in the treatment of pain from rheumatoid arthritis and osteoarthritis, or from the spinal disorder ankylosing spondylitis. It is not recommended for children.

▲ side-effects: there may be a skin rash; rarely, there is an allergic response or gastrointestinal bleeding.

● warning: flurbiprofen should not be administered to patients who are suffering from gastric or intestinal bleeding (as with a peptic ulcer); who are pregnant or lactating; who are allergic to aspirin or other anti-inflammatory drugs; who have reduced kidney function; who are asthmatic; or who are already taking aspirin, an anticoagulant or a drug to control the blood level of glucose.
Related article: FROBEN.

fluspirilene is an ANTIPSYCHOTIC drug of the diphenylbutylpiperidine class used to treat psychosis (such as schizophrenia). It is also available as an aqueous suspension for intramuscular injection, potency lasting between 5 and 15 days.
▲ side-effects: extrapyramidal motor disorders are commonly seen with high doses about 48 hours after injection, with abnormal movements, restlessness and tremor. There may be drowsiness, pallor and hypothermia, insomnia, depression and, frequently, restlessness and sweating. Rashes and jaundice may occur, and there may be dry mouth, constipation, difficulty in urination, and blurred vision. Prolonged usage may cause tissue damage (in the form of nodules) at the site of injection.
● warning: fluspirilene should be administered only with extreme caution to patients who suffer from heart or vascular disease, from kidney or liver disease, from parkinsonism, from epilepsy, or from depression; or who are pregnant or lactating. Dosage should be reduced for the elderly; it is not suitable for children.
Related article: REDEPTIN.

fluvoxamine maleate is an ANTIDEPRESSANT drug used to treat depressive illness. It has the advantage over some other antidepressant drugs in that it works by inhibiting uptake of the neurotransmitter SEROTONIN, and so has relatively less sedative side effects, though it may have gastointestinal actions. It is available as tablets.
▲ side-effects: it may impair performance of skilled tasks such as driving; may cause a rash (if so discontinue treatment), convulsions, headache, tremor, nausea, vomiting, and diarrhoea (which may be severe). It may enhance the effects of alcohol.
● warning: it should not be given to epileptics, and it should be given with caution to patients with liver or kidney damage, and those who have diabetes, or who are pregnant. It should be avoided in lactating women. MAO inhibitor anti-depressant drugs should not be used until at least five weeks after discontinuing fluvoxamine maleate.
Related article: FAVERIN.

Formulix (*Cilag*) is a proprietary compound ANALGESIC, available only on prescription to private patients, used as a painkiller. Produced in the form of tablets, it is a preparation of the OPIATE codeine phosphate and the non-narcotic analgesic paracetamol that contains more codeine than the usual compound preparation known as CO-CODAMOL, and is not recommended for children under 3 years of age. The preparation is in the form of an elixir.
▲/● side-effects/warning: *see* CODEINE PHOSPHATE; PARACETAMOL.

Fortral (*Sterling Research*) is a proprietary, NARCOTIC ANALGESIC, a controlled drug, which is not available from the National Health Service. Produced in the form of tablets, capsules, ampoules for injection, and anal suppositories, its active constituent is the OPIATE pentazocine. Fortral suppositories are not recommended for children; as tablets and capsules Fortral is not recommended for children aged under 6 years; and as injections Fortral is not recommended for children aged under 12 months.
▲/ ⬣ side-effects/warning: *see* PENTAZOCINE.

Fortunan (*Allen & Hanburys*) is a proprietary, ANTIPSYCHOTIC drug, available only on prescription, used as a major TRANQUILLIZER to treat patients with behavioural disturbances, or who are psychotic, particularly schizophrenic. It may be used in the short term to treat severe anxiety. Produced in the form of tablets (in five strengths), Fortunan is a preparation of haloperidol.
▲/ ⬣ side-effects/warning: *see* HALOPERIDOL.

Frisium (*Hoechst*) is a proprietary form of the BENZODIAZEPINE clobazam, used primarily as an ANXIOLYTIC to treat anxiety, nervous tension and restlessness. It may also be used to assist in the treatment of epilepsy. Available on prescription only to private patients, Frisium is produced in the form of capsules. It is not recommended for children aged under 3 years.
▲/ ⬣ side-effects/warning: *see* CLOBAZAM.

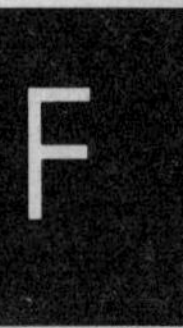

Froben (*Boots*) is a proprietary, non-steroid, non-narcotic ANALGESIC available only on prescription, used to relieve pain – particularly arthritic and rheumatic pain – and to treat other musculo-skeletal disorders. Its active constituent is flurbiprofen, and it is produced in the form of tablets, as sustained-release capsules (Froben SR), and as anal suppositories. Not recommended for children, Froben should not be administered to patients with a peptic ulcer or gastrointestinal bleeding; special care is necessary in the treatment of patients who are pregnant or lactating; whose kidneys are not fully functional; or who have asthma.
▲/ ⬣ side-effects/warning: *see* FLURBIPROFEN.

Galcodine (*Galen*) is a proprietary ANTITUSSIVE, available only on prescription, used to encourage the loosening of a dry, painful cough. Produced in the form of an orange-flavoured sugar-free linctus (in two strengths, the weaker under the name Galcodine Paediatric) for dilution (the potency of the dilute linctus is retained for 14 days), galcodine is a preparation of the OPIATE codeine phosphate. It is not recommended for children aged under 12 months.
▲/ ♣ side-effects/warning: *see* CODEINE PHOSPHATE.

Galenphol (*Galen*) is a proprietary cough suppressant (ANTITUSSIVE), available only on prescription, used to encourage the loosening of a dry, painful cough. Produced in the form of an aniseed-flavoured sugar-free linctus (in three strengths, the weakest under the name Galenphol Linctus Paediatric, the strongest under the name Galenphol Linctus Strong) for dilution (the potency of the dilute linctus is retained for 14 days), Galenphol is a preparation of the OPIATE pholcodine.
▲/ ♣ side-effects/warning: *see* PHOLCODINE.

Gamanil (*Merck*) is a proprietary, TRICYCLIC ANTIDEPRESSANT drug, available only on prescription, used to treat depressive illness and associated symptoms. Produced in the form of tablets, Gamanil represents a preparation of lofepramine hydrochloride. It is not recommended for children.
▲/ ♣ side-effects/warning: *see* LOFEPRAMINE.

Gardenal sodium (*May & Baker*) is a proprietary form of the ANTICONVULSANT BARBITURATE phenobarbitone, and is on the controlled drugs list. Produced in vials for injection, it is used to treat several forms of epilepsy including generalized tonic-clonic and partial seizures, although it should be administered with extreme caution to children or the elderly.
▲/ ♣ side-effects/warning: *see* PHENOBARBITONE.

Gastrobid Continus (*Napp*) is a proprietary ANTINAUSEANT and ANTI-EMETIC, used to treat digestive disturbances resulting in nausea; and for nausea, severe indigestion and vomiting after radiation or cytotoxic drug therapy. Available only on prescription, the active constituent, metoclopramide hydrochloride, works by reducing nausea and vomiting and allowing the passage of absorbable nutrients in food in the stomach down into the intestines. It is produced in the form of sustained-release tablets. It is not recommended for patients less than 20 years of age.
▲/ ♣ side-effects/warning: *see* METOCLOPRAMIDE.

Gastromax (*Farmitalia Carlo Erba*) is a proprietary ANTINAUSEANT and ANTI-EMETIC, used to treat digestive disturbances resulting in nausea; and for nausea, severe indigestion and vomiting after radiation or cytotoxic drug therapy. Available only on prescription, the active constituent, metoclopramide hydrochloride, works by reducing nausea and vomiting and allowing the passage of absorbable nutrients in food in the stomach down into the intestines. It is produced in the form of sustained-release capsules. It is not recommended for patients less than 20 years of age.
▲/ ♣ side-effects/warning: *see* METOCLOPRAMIDE.

Gee's linctus is a less formal name for the (ANTITUSSIVE) non-proprietary, opiate squill cough linctus.
see OPIATE SQUILL LINCTUS AND PASTILLES.

Gee's pastilles is a less formal name for the (ANTITUSSIVE) non-proprietary, opiate squill cough pastilles.
see OPIATE SQUILL LINCTUS AND PASTILLES.

***general anaesthetic**: *see* ANAESTHETIC.

G

H

Haldol (*Janssen*) is a proprietary form of the powerful ANTIPSYCHOTIC drug haloperidol. Available only on prescription, it is used to treat and tranquillize psychosis (such as schizophrenia), in which it is particularly suitable for treating manic forms of behavioural disturbance. It may be used alternatively to treat severe anxiety in the short term, as a premedication before surgery, or to control patients in delirium tremens or with alcohol withdrawal problems. Haldol is produced in the form of tablets (in two strengths), as a liquid to take orally (in two strengths, under the name Haldol Oral Liquid), and in ampoules for injection.

▲/● side-effects/warning: *see* HALOPERIDOL.

Haldol Decanoate (*Janssen*) is another form of HALDOL, available only on prescription, it is an ANTIPSYCHOTIC used to treat forms of psychosis on a long-term maintenance basis. Its active constituent is the decanoate salt of haloperidol. Produced in ampoules (in two strengths) for injection, it is not recommended for children.

▲/● side-effects/warning: *see* HALOPERIDOL.

haloperidol is an ANTIPSYCHOTIC drug of the butyrophenone class used to treat psychosis (such as schizophrenia), in which it is particularly suitable for treating manic forms of behavioural disturbance, especially in order to effect emergency control. The drug may also be used to treat severe anxiety in the short term. It may also be employed as an ANTI-EMETIC for vomiting resulting from chemotherapy treatment. It has shown to be of value in the treatment of minor tics and intractable hiccup. Administration is oral in the form of capsules, tablets, a liquid or an elixir, or by injection (which may be short-acting or 'depot').

▲ side-effects: patients should be warned before treatment that their judgement and powers of concentration may become defective under treatment. Extrapyramidal motor symptoms (muscle spasms, tremor) are common with high dosage and prolonged use may cause tardive dyskinesias. There may be restlessness, insomnia and nightmares; rashes and jaundice may occur; and there may be dry mouth, gastrointestinal disturbance, difficulties in urinating, and blurred vision. Rarely, there is weight loss and impaired kidney function.

● warning: haloperidol should not be administered to patients who suffer from a reduction in the bone-marrow's capacity to produce blood cells. It should be administered only with caution to those with heart or vascular disease, kidney or liver disease, parkinsonism, or depression; or who are pregnant or lactating. It is not recommended for children.

Related articles: DOZIC; FORTUNAN; HALDOL; HALDOL DECANOATE; SERENACE.

halothane is a powerful general ANAESTHETIC that is widely used both for induction and for maintenance of anaesthesia during surgical operations. Used in combination with oxygen or nitrous oxide-oxygen mixtures, halothane vapour is non-irritant and even pleasant to inhale, does not induce coughing, and seldom causes post-operative vomiting. Administration is through a calibrated vaporizer in order to control concentration.

▲ side-effects: there may be liver damage. Repetition of anaesthesia by halothane is inadvisable within 3 months.

◆ warning: halothane causes a slowing of the heart rate and shallowness of breathing; both must be monitored during anaesthesia to prevent high levels of carbon dioxide or dangerously slow pulse and low blood pressure. The vapour is not good as a muscle relaxant, and muscle relaxants may have to be used in addition during specific types of surgery.
Related article: FLUOTHANE.

Hedex (*Sterling Health*) is a proprietary, non-prescription, non-narcotic ANALGESIC produced in the form of tablets and as a soluble powder. It contains paracetamol.
▲/◆ side-effects/warning: *see* PARACETAMOL.

Hedex Plus (*Sterling Health*) is a proprietary, non-prescription combination ANALGESIC produced in the form of capsules. It contains paracetamol, caffeine and codeine.
▲/◆ side-effects/warning: *see* CAFFEINE; CODEINE; PARACETAMOL.

Heminevrin (*Astra*) is a proprietary SEDATIVE and ANTICONVULSANT, available only on prescription, used to treat insomnia, states of confusion or agitation in the elderly, and (under rigorous monitoring) acute alcohol withdrawal symptoms. It may also be used as an intravenous infusion for the control of convulsions in status epilepticus. Produced in the form of capsules, as a sugar-free syrup for dilution (the potency of the syrup once dilute is retained for 14 days), and in flasks (bottles) for intravenous infusion, Heminevrin is a preparation of chlormethiazole. Not recommended for children.
▲/◆ side-effects/warning: *see* CHLORMETHIAZOLE.

heroin is a more familiar term for the NARCOTIC ANALGESIC drug diamorphine.
see DIAMORPHINE.

Histalix (*Wallace*) is a proprietary, non-prescription expectorant and ANTITUSSIVE, which is not available from the National Health Service. Produced in the form of a syrup, its active constituents include ammonium chloride, sodium citrate, DIPHENHYDRAMINE HYDROCHLORIDE and menthol.

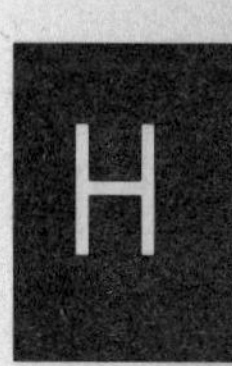

***hormones** are body substances produced and secreted by glands into the bloodstream. They are carried to certain organs and cells, which carry specific receptors for the hormones, and on which the hormones have specific effect. The major classes of hormones include: adrenocorticosteroids, produced mainly in the cortex of adrenal glands; ADRENALINE and NORADRENALINE, from the medulla of the adrenal gland; thyroid hormones, produced by the thyroid gland; the sex hormones oestrogens and androgens, produced mainly by the ovaries or the testes; the pancreatic hormones (e.g. insulin); and the hormones that cause secretion or production of these hormones, e.g. gonadotrophin-releasing hormone. Hormone preparations (sometimes in synthetic form) can often be administered therapeutically to alleviate hormone deficiency states.

Hydergine (*Sandoz*) is a proprietary form of the cerebral VASODILATOR drug co-dergocrine mesylate, used primarily to assist in the management of elderly patients with mild to moderate dementia. Hydergine is thought to work by enhancing blood flow to the brain. Available only on prescription, it is produced in the form of tablets (in two strengths), and is not recommended for children.

▲/● side-effects/warning: *see* CODERGOCRINE MESYLATE.

hydroxyzine hydrochloride is an ANXIOLYTIC drug, an ANTIHISTAMINE used to treat anxiety. Administration is oral in the form of tablets or as a syrup.

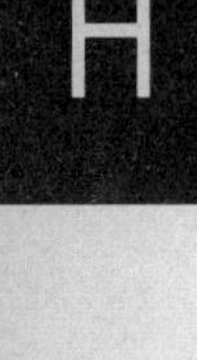

▲ side-effects: drowsiness is fairly common; there is sometimes also neural dysfunction and, with high doses, involuntary movements, dizziness and confusion.

● warning: hydroxyzine hydrochloride should not be administered to patients who are pregnant or who are alcoholic, and should be used with caution to patients with kidney damage; all patients should be warned prior to treatment that their speed of thought and reaction may be impaired by treatment.
Related article: ATARAX.

hyoscine, also known as scopolamine (in the USA), is a powerful alkaloid drug derived from plants of the belladonna family. By itself it is an effective SEDATIVE and HYPNOTIC – it is often used together with the OPIATE papaveretum as a premedication prior to surgery – and an ANTI-EMETIC (in which capacity it is found in travel-sickness medications). Administration is oral in the form of tablets or by injection.

▲ side-effects: there may be drowsiness, dizziness and dry mouth; sometimes there is also blurred vision and difficulty in urinating.

● warning: hyoscine (or its bromide salts) should not be administered to patients with glaucoma; it should be administered with caution to those with heart or intestinal disease, or urinary retention, or who are elderly.
Related articles: JOY-RIDES; KWELLS; OMNOPON-SCOPOLAMINE; SCOPODERM TTS.

Hypnomidate (*Janssen*) is a proprietary general ANAESTHETIC used primarily for initial induction of anaesthesia. Available only on prescription, it is produced in ampoules for injection (in two strengths, the stronger for dilution), and is a preparation of etomidate. It should not be allowed to come into contact with plastic equipment.

▲/● side-effects/warning: *see* ETOMIDATE.

***hypnotics** are a type of drug that induce sleep by direct action on various centres of the brain. They are used mainly to treat insomnia. The most used hypnotics are the BENZODIAZEPINES (e.g diazepam and nitrazepam), which are safer than using derivatives of chloral (e.g. chloral hydrate) or the BARBITURATES (e.g. amylobarbitone), which may cause dependence (addiction). Some hypnotics may cause a hangover effect on waking in the mornings and psychological dependence may become problem.

Hypnovel is a proprietary preparation of the powerful BENZODIAZEPINE midazolam, available only on prescription, used mainly for sedation, particularly as a premedication prior to surgery, for the initial induction of anaesthesia, or for the short-term anaesthesia required for endoscopy or minor surgical examinations. Its effect is often accompanied by a form of amnesia. It is produced in ampoules for infusion (in two strengths).

▲/● side-effects/warning: *see* MIDAZOLAM

Hypon (*Calmic*) is a proprietary, non-prescription compound ANALGESIC preparation, which is not available from the National Health Service. Produced in the form of tablets, Hypon is a combination of aspirin, the STIMULANT caffeine, and the OPIATE codeine phosphate. It is not recommended for children.
▲/ ✚ side-effects/warning: *see* ASPIRIN; CAFFEINE; CODEINE PHOSPHATE.

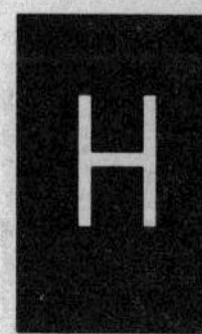

Ibufhalal (*Halal Parmaceuticals*) is a proprietary, non-narcotic, ANALGESIC containing ibuprofen, which also has ANTI-INFLAMMATORY properties (NSAID). It is available without prescription as tablets (in three strengths).

▲/● side-effects/warning: *see* IBUPROFEN.

Ibular (*Lagap*) is a proprietary, ANTI-INFLAMMATORY, non-narcotic ANALGESIC, available only on prescription, used to treat the pain of rheumatic and other musculo-skeletal disorders. Produced in the form of tablets, Ibular is a preparation of ibuprofen.

▲/● side-effects/warning: *see* IBUPROFEN.

ibuprofen is a non-steroidal, ANTI-INFLAMMATORY, non-narcotic ANALGESIC drug used primarily to treat the pain of rheumatism and other musculo-skeletal disorders, but also used sometimes to treat other forms of pain, including menstrual pain. In its anti-inflammatory capacity it is not as powerful as some other drugs, however, and dosage tends to be high to compensate. Administration is oral in the form of tablets or sustained-release capsules, or as a syrup.

▲ side-effects: administration with or following meals reduces the risk of gastrointestinal disturbance and nausea. There may be headache, dizziness and ringing in the ears (tinnitus), and some patients experience sensitivity reactions or blood disorders. Occasionally, there is fluid retention.

● warning: ibuprofen should be administered with caution to patients with impaired liver or kidney function, gastric ulcers, or severe allergies (including asthma), or who are pregnant.

Related articles: APSIFEN; BRUFEN; EBUFAC; EFUFAC; FENBID; IBUFAHAL; IBULAR; INOVEN: LIDIFEN; MICROFEN; MOTRIN; NUROFEN; PACIFENE; PAXOFEN; PROFLEX; RELCOFEN.

Imbrilon (*Berk*) is a proprietary, ANTI-INFLAMMATORY, non-narcotic ANALGESIC, available only on prescription, used to treat the pain of rheumatic and other musculo-skeletal disorders (including gout). Produced in the form of capsules (in two strengths), and as anal suppositories, Imbrilon is a preparation of indomethacin. It is not recommended for children.

▲/● side-effects/warning: *see* INDOMETHACIN.

imipramine is a TRICYCLIC ANTIDEPRESSANT drug, which has fewer sedative properties than many others. It is thus suited more to the treatment of withdrawn and apathetic patients than to those who are agitated and restless. As is the case with many such drugs, imipramine can also be used to treat bedwetting at night by children (aged over 7 years). Administration is oral in the form of tablets or as a syrup, or by injection.

▲ side-effects: common effects include sedation (affecting driving ability), dry mouth and blurred vision; there may also be difficulty in urinating, sweating and irregular heartbeat, behavioural disturbances, a rash, a state of confusion, and/or a loss of libido. Rarely, there are also blood disorders.

● warning: imipramine should not be administered to patients who suffer from heart disease or psychosis; it should be administered with caution to patients who suffer from diabetes, epilepsy, liver or thyroid disease, glaucoma or

urinary retention; or who are pregnant or lactating. Withdrawal of treatment must be gradual.
Related article: TOFRANIL.

Inderal (*ICI*) is a proprietary BETA-BLOCKER, available only on prescription, used to treat anxiety (ANXIOLYTIC) and to try to prevent migraine attacks (ANTIMIGRAINE). Produced in the form of tablets (in four strengths), and in ampoules for injection; as sustained-release capsules (in two strengths, Inderal LA and the weaker Half-Inderal LA), and as tablets (in five strengths). Inderal is a preparation of propranolol hydrochloride.
▲/ ✚ side-effects/warning: *see* PROPRANOLOL.

Indian hemp is the name of the plant from which the psychedelic drug cannabis is prepared.
see CANNABIS.

Indocid (*Morson*) is a proprietary, ANTI-INFLAMMATORY, non-narcotic ANALGESIC, available only on prescription, used to treat the pain of rheumatic and other musculo-skeletal disorders (including gout and degenerative bone diseases). Produced in the form of capsules (in two strengths), and as sustained-release capsules (under the name Indocid-R), as anal suppositories, and as a sugar-free suspension, Indocid is a preparation of indomethacin. It is not recommended for children.
▲/ ✚ side-effects/warning: *see* INDOMETHACIN.

Indoflex (*Unimed*) is a proprietary, ANTI-INFLAMMATORY ANALGESIC, available only on prescription, used to treat the pain of rheumatic and other musculo-skeletal disorders (including gout and degenerative bone diseases). Produced in the form of capsules, Indoflex is a preparation of indomethacin. It is not recommended for children.
▲/ ✚ side-effects/warning: *see* INDOMETHACIN.

Indolar SR (*Lagap*) is a proprietary form of the non-steroidal, ANTI-INFLAMMATORY, non-narcotic ANALGESIC indomethacin. It is available on prescription, as sustained-release tablets (in two strengths), to treat pain and inflammation associated with musculo-skeletal disorders, such as rheumatic disease.
▲/ ✚ side-effects/warning: *see* INDOMETHACIN.

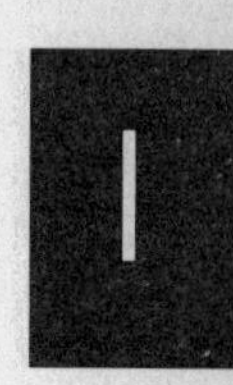

indomethacin is a non-steroidal, ANTI-INFLAMMATORY, non-narcotic ANALGESIC drug used to treat rheumatic and muscular pain caused by inflammation and/or bone degeneration particularly at the joints. It is also used to treat menstrual pain (dysmenorrhea). Administration is mostly oral in the form of tablets, capsules, sustained-release capsules or as a liquid, but its use in anal suppositories is especially effective for the relief of pain overnight and stiffness in the morning. Some proprietary preparations are not recommended for children.
▲ side-effects: all drugs of this type are prone to give gastro-intestinal discomfort. During treatment, concentration and speed of reaction may be affected; there may also be headache and dizziness, although further mental effects (including depression and confusion) are rare. Some patients experience ringing in the ears (tinnitus) blood disorders, and high blood pressure (hypertension). There may be visual disturbances, tingling in the toes and fingertips and (following the use of suppositories) anal itching.

- ● warning: indomethacin should not be administered to patients who suffer from peptic ulcers or who are sensitive to aspirin. It should be administered with caution to those who suffer from allergic conditions (such as asthma), from epilepsy, from psychological disturbances, or from impaired function of the liver or kidneys, who are elderly, or who are pregnant. Blood counts and ophthalmic checks are advised during prolonged treatment. Suppositories should not be used by patients with anorectal infections or piles (haemorrhoids).
  Related articles: ARTRACIN; FLEXIS CONTINUS; IMBRILON; INDOCID; INDOLAR SR; INDOFLEX; INDOLAR SR; INDOMOD; MOBILAN; SLO-INDO.

Indomod (*Benzon*) is a proprietary, ANTI-INFLAMMATORY, non-narcotic ANALGESIC, available only on prescription, used to treat the pain of rheumatic and other musculo-skeletal disorders (including gout, bursitis and tendonitis). Produced in the form of sustained-release capsules (in two strengths), Indomod is a preparation of indomethacin. It is not recommended for children.
▲/● side-effects/warning: *see* INDOMETHACIN.

Inoven (*Janssen*) is a proprietary, non-narcotic, ANALGESIC containing ibuprofen, which also has ANTI-INFLAMMATORY properties (NSAID). It is available without prescription as tablets (in three strengths).
▲/● side-effects/warning: *see* IBUPROFEN.

Integrin (*Sterling Research*) is a powerful ANTIPSYCHOTIC drug, available only on prescription, used to treat and tranquillize patients who are undergoing behavioural disturbances (states of both apathetic withdrawal and hyperactive mania), or who are psychotic (particularly schizophrenic). It is also used to treat severe anxiety in the short term. Produced in the form of capsules and tablets, Integrin is a preparation of the antipsychotic drug oxypertine. It is not recommended for children.
▲/● side-effects/warning: *see* OXYPERTINE.

Ionamin (*Lipha*) is a proprietary preparation of the STIMULANT drug phentermine used, in the short term only, to assist in the medical treatment of obesity. On the controlled drugs list, Ionamin is produced in the form of sustained-release capsules (in two strengths). It is not recommended for children aged under 6 years.
▲/● side-effects/warning: *see* PHENTERMINE.

iprindole is a TRICYCLIC ANTIDEPRESSANT drug of a type that has fewer sedative properties than many others. In the treatment of depressive illness it is thus suited more to the treatment of withdrawn and apathetic patients than to those who are agitated and restless. Administration is oral in the form of tablets.

- ▲ side-effects: common effects include sedation (affecting driving ability), dry mouth and blurred vision; there may also be difficulty in urinating, sweating and irregular heartbeat, behavioural disturbances, a rash, a state of confusion, and/or a loss of libido. Rarely, there are also blood disorders.
- ● warning: iprindole should not be administered to patients who suffer from heart disease or psychosis; it should be administered with caution to

patients who suffer from diabetes, epilepsy, liver or thyroid disease, glaucoma or urinary retention; or who are pregnant or lactating. Withdrawal of treatment must be gradual.
Related article: PRONDOL.

isoaminile citrate is a drug that suppresses a cough (ANTITUSSIVE); such drugs are used medically only when absolutely necessary, and when sputum retention is guaranteed to do no harm. Administration is oral in the form of a linctus.
▲ side-effects: constipation is often associated with treatment.
● warning: isoaminile citrate should not be administered to patients with any impairment of airflow in the respiratory passages (as in asthma), or who would find sputum retention a hazard (as in chronic bronchitis).
Related article: DIMYRIL; ISOAMINILE LINCTUS.

isoaminile linctus is a non-proprietary preparation of isoaminile citrate, available only on prescription, used only under specific circumstances to treat a dry or persistent and painful cough (ANTITUSSIVE). It is produced in the form of a syrup for dilution (the potency of the syrup once dilute is retained for 14 days).
▲/● side-effects/warning: *see* ISOAMINILE CITRATE.

isocarboxazid is an ANTI-DEPRESSANT drug, an MAO INHIBITOR (mono amine oxidase inhibitor, or MAOI) used accordingly to treat depressive illness. Administration is oral in the form of tablets. It is not suitable for children.
▲ side-effects: dizziness is fairly common. There may also be headache, dry mouth, blurred vision and tremor; some patients experience constipation and difficulty in urinating; a rash may break out. Susceptible patients may undergo psychotic episodes.
● warning: isocarboxazid should not be administered to patients with disease of the liver or the blood vessels, or epilepsy. Treatment with this drug requires the strict avoidance of certain foods (particularly cheese, pickled fish, yeast or meat extracts), some beverages and of certain other medications, such as 'cold-cures'; professional counselling on this subject is essential. Withdrawal of treatment should be gradual.
Related article: MARPLAN.

isoflurane is a general ANAESTHETIC related to ENFLURANE, produced as a gas to be used in solution with oxygen or nitrous oxide-oxygen. Administration is through a specially calibrated vaporiser. It is used particularly for the initial induction of anaesthesia.
▲ side-effects: there may be an increase in heart rate accompanied by a fall in blood pressure (especially in younger patients).
● warning: treatment depresses respiration. The drug also produces muscle relaxation, and/or enhances the effect of muscle-relaxant drugs administered simultaneously.
Related article: ISOFLURANE.

Isoflurane (*Abbott*) is a proprietary form of the general ANAESTHETIC isoflurane.
▲/● side-effects/warning: *see* ISOFLURANE.

isometheptene mucate is an ANTIMIGRAINE drug used in combination with a sedative (such as dichloralphenazone) to treat

ISOMETHEPTENE MUCATE

migraine attacks. Administration is oral in the form of capsules.

▲ side-effects: there may be dizziness associated with peripheral disturbances in blood circulation.

● warning: the combination should not be administered to patients with glaucoma; it should be administered with caution to those with cardiovascular disease, or those on MAO INHIBITOR therapy.

Related article: MIDRID.

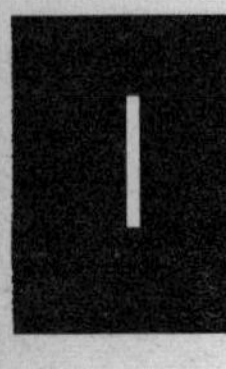

Joy-Rides (*Stafford-Miller*) is a proprietary, non-prescription, ANTI-EMETIC ANTICHOLINERGIC formulation for the treatment of motion sickness. It contains the atropine-like drug hyoscine.
▲/ ✚ side-effects/warning: *see* HYOSCINE.

Junifen (*Boots*) is a proprietary, non-narcotic ANALGESIC, which has valuable additional ANTI-INFLAMMATORY properties. Available only on prescription, Junifen is used to relieve fever and moderate pain in children. It is produced in the form of a suspension for taking by mouth. It is a preparation of ibuprofen. Not recommended for children under one year.
▲/ ✚ side-effects/warning: *see* IBUPROFEN.

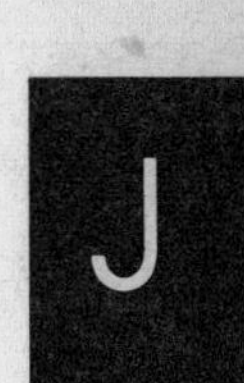

Kemadrin (*Wellcome*) is a proprietary preparation of the ANTICHOLINERGIC procyclidine hydrochloride, available only on prescription, used in the treatment of parkinsonism and to control tremors within drug-induced states involving involuntary movement (*see* ANTIPARKINSONIAN). Produced in the form of tablets and in ampoules for injection, Kemadrin is not recommended for children.
▲/ ♦ side-effects/warning: *see* PROCYCLIDINE.

K

Ketalar (*Parke-Davis*) is a proprietary preparation of the general ANAESTHETIC ketamine, in the form of ketamine chloride. Available only on prescription, Ketalar is produced as vials for injection (in three strengths).
▲/ ♦ side-effects/warning: *see* KETAMINE.

ketamine is a general ANAESTHETIC that is used mainly for surgery on children, in whom hallucinogenic side-effects seem to appear less often than in adults. Ketamine has a good reputation for increasing muscle tone, maintaining good air passage, and having fair analgesic qualities in doses too low for actual anaesthesia (and the hallucinations can be avoided through the simultaneous use of other drugs). Administration is either by intramuscular injection or by intravenous infusion.
▲ side-effects: transient hallucinations may occur. Recovery is relatively slow.
♦ warning: ketamine should not be administered to patients who suffer from high blood pressure (hypertension) or who are prone to hallucinations.
Related article: KETALAR.

ketoprofen is a non-steroid, ANTI-INFLAMMATORY, non-narcotic ANALGESIC drug, used to treat rheumatic and muscular pain caused by inflammation, and to treat gout. It is produced in the form of capsules, anal suppositories and for injection. The drug should be taken with food in order to avoid possible gastrointestinal upset.
▲ side-effects: there may be gastrointestinal upset; hypersensitivity reactions; suppositories may cause irritation.
♦ warning: use with caution in the presence of gastric ulceration, liver or kidney damage, allergic disorders or pregnancy. It tends to enhance the effect of anticoagulant drugs. Dosage should be closely monitored.
Related articles: ALRHEUMAT; ORUDIS; ORUVAIL.

Kwells (*Nicholas-Kiwi*) is a proprietary, ANTCHOLINERGIC ANTI-EMETIC, non-prescription, anti-motion sickness preparation containing hyoscine.
▲/ ♦ side-effects/warning: *see* HYOSCINE.

Labiton (*L A B*) is a proprietary, non-prescription tonic, which is not available from the National Health Service. Used primarily to stimulate the appetite, Labiton contains the STIMULANT caffeine, vitamin B in the form of thiamine, extract of kola nut, and ethyl alcohol. It is not recommended for children.

♣ warning: labiton should not be taken by patients who are already taking drugs that directly affect the central nervous system, or who have liver disease.

Laboprin (*L A B*) is a proprietary, non-prescription preparation of the non-narcotic ANALGESIC aspirin, which is not available from the National Health Service. Produced in the form of tablets, Laboprin also contains the essential amino acid lysine. It is not recommended for children.

▲/♣ side-effects/warning: *see* ASPIRIN.

Laraflex (*Lagap*) is a proprietary, non-steroidal, ANTI-INFLAMMATORY non-narcotic ANALGESIC, available only on prescription, used to relieve pain – particularly rheumatic and arthritic pain – and to treat other musculo-skeletal disorders. Its active constituent is naproxen, and it is produced in the form of tablets (in two strengths). Not recommended for children.

▲/♣ side-effects/warning: *see* NAPROXEN.

Larapam (*Lagap*) is a proprietary, non-steroidal, ANTI-INFLAMMATORY non-narcotic ANALGESIC, available only on prescription, used to relieve pain – particularly rheumatic and arthritic pain – and to treat other musculo-skeletal disorders. Its active constituent is piroxicam, and it is produced in the form of tablets (in two strengths). Not recommended for children.

▲/♣ side-effects/warning: *see* PIROXICAM.

Largactil (*May & Baker*) is a proprietary preparation of the PHENOTHIAZINE ANTIPSYCHOTIC drug chlorpromazine hydrochloride, used primarily to treat patients who are undergoing behavioural disturbances (as a major TRANQUILLIZER), or who are psychotic particularly schizophrenic. It is also used to treat severe anxiety, or as an ANTI-EMETIC sedative prior to surgery. Available only on prescription, Largactil is produced in the form of tablets (in three strengths), as a syrup (under the name Largactil Syrup), as a suspension (under the name Largactil Forte Suspension), as anal suppositories (under the name Largactil Suppositories), and in ampoules for injection (under the name Largactil Injection). In the form of the suppositories and the ampoules for injection Largactil is not recommended for use with children.

▲/♣ side-effects/warning: *see* CHLORPROMAZINE.

Larodopa (*Roche*) is a proprietary form of the powerful drug levodopa, used in ANTIPARKINSONIAN treatment. It is particularly good at relieving the rigidity and slowness of movement associated with the disease, although it does not always improve the tremor. Produced in the form of tablets, Larodopa is not recommended for children.

▲/♣ side-effects/warning: *see* LEVODOPA.

Lederfen (*Lederle*) is a proprietary, non-steroid, ANTI-INFLAMMATORY non-narcotic ANALGESIC, available only on prescription, used to relieve pain – particularly rheumatic and

arthritic pain – and to treat other musculo-skeletal disorders. Its active constituent is fenbufen, and it is produced in the form of tablets (in two strengths), capsules (under the name Lederfen Capsules), and as effervescent tablets (Lederfen F). Not recommended for children.
▲/ ✚ side-effects/warning: *see* FENBUFEN.

L

Lem-sip (*Nicholas-Kiwi*) is a proprietary, non-prescription cold relief preparation containing the non-narcotic ANALGESIC paracetamol, the SYMPATHOMIMETIC phenylephrine, sodium citrate and ascorbic acid.
▲/ ✚ side-effects/warning: *see* PARACETAMOL.

Lentizol (*Parke-Davis*) is a proprietary, TRICYCLIC ANTIDEPRESSANT, available only on prescription, used to treat depressive illness, and particularly in cases where some degree of sedation is called for. Produced in the form of capsules (in two strengths), Lentizol is a preparation of amitriptyline hydrochloride, and is not recommended for children.
▲/ ✚ side-effects/warning: *see* AMITRIPTYLINE.

levodopa is an immensely powerful ANTIPARKINSONIAN drug used to treat parkinsonism (but not the symptoms of parkinsonism induced by drugs). It works by conversion into the neurotransmitter DOPAMINE within the brain. Effective in reducing the slowness of movement and rigidity associated with parkinsonism, levodopa is not so successful in controlling the tremor. Administration is in the form of capsules or tablets, often combined with another form of drug that inhibits the conversion of levodopa to dopamine outside the brain. It is the presence of such an inhibitor that may produce involuntary movements. Initial dosage should be minimal and increased gradually; intervals between doses may be critical to each individual patient. Treated with levodopa a patient may be expected to improve quality of life for 6 to 18 months, and for that improvement to obtain for up to another 2 years; thereafter a slow decline is to be expected.
▲ side-effects: there may be nausea, dizziness, agitation, anorexia, irregularity of the heart rate, insomnia and restlessness, and discoloration of the urine. Psychiatric symptoms and involuntary movements may direct dosage quantities.
✚ warning: levodopa should not be administered to patients with a specific form of glaucoma (closed-angle); it should be administered with caution to those with heart disease, psychiatric illness, diabetes mellitus or peptic ulcers. Monitoring of heart, blood, liver and kidney functions is advisable during prolonged treatment; some check on psychological disposition should also be made.
Related articles: BROCADOPA; LARODOPA; MADOPAR; SINEMET.

Lexotan (*Roche*) is a proprietary ANXIOLYTIC drug, available on prescription only to private patients, used to treat anxiety in the short term. Produced in the form of tablets (in two strengths), Lexotan is a preparation of the BENZODIAZEPINE bromazepam. It is not recommended for children.
▲/ ✚ side-effects/warning: *see* BROMAZEPAM.

Librium (*Roche*) is a proprietary form of the BENZODIAZEPINE chlordiazepoxide, used as an

ANXIOLYTIC to treat anxiety, insomnia in the short term, and symptoms of acute alcohol withdrawal. Available on prescription only to private patients, Librium is produced in the form of tablets (in three strengths), capsules (in two strengths) and powder for reconstitution as a medium for injection. It is not recommended for children.

▲/● side-effects/warning: *see* CHLORDIAZEPOXIDE.

Lidifen (*Berk*) is a proprietary form of the non-steroidal, ANTI-INFLAMMATORY, ANALGESIC drug ibuprofen. Available on prescription it is used to treat pain and inflammation, particularly caused by musculo-skeletal disorders. Administration is in the form of tablets (in 3 strengths).

▲/● side-effects/warning: *see* IBUPROFEN.

lignocaine is primarily a local ANAESTHETIC, the medium of choice for very many topical or minor surgical procedures, especially in dentistry (because it is absorbed directly through mucous membranes). It is, for example, used on the throat to prepare a patient for bronchoscopy. For general anaesthesia it may be combined with adrenaline. But it is also administered in the treatment of heart conditions involving heartbeat irregularities, and is effective in safely slowing the heart rate (particularly after a heart attack). Administration is (in the form of a solution of lignocaine hydrochloride) by infiltration, injection or infusion, or topically as a gel, an ointment, a spray, a lotion, or as eye-drops.

▲ side-effects: there is generally a slowing of the heart rate and a fall in blood pressure. Some patients under anaesthetic become agitated, others enter a state of euphoria.

● warning: lignocaine should not be administered to patients with the neuromuscular disease myasthenia gravis; it should be administered with caution to those with heart or liver failure (in order not to cause depression of the central nervous system and convulsions), or from epilepsy. Dosage should be reduced for the elderly and the debilitated. Full facilities for emergency cardio-respiratory resuscitation should be on hand during anaesthetic treatment.

Related article: XYLOTOX.

Limbitrol (*Roche*) is a proprietary compound ANTIDEPRESSANT, available on prescription only to private patients, used to treat depressive illness and associated anxiety. Produced in capsules (in two strengths, under the names Limbitrol 5 and Limbitrol 10), Limbitrol's active constituents are amitriptyline and chlordiazepoxide. It is not recommended for the elderly or for children.

▲/● side-effects/warning: *see* AMITRIPTYLINE; CHLORDIAZEPOXIDE.

Lingraine (*Winthrop*) is a proprietary ANTIMIGRAINE drug, available only on prescription. Produced in the form of tablets, Lingraine is a preparation of the ergot-derived alkaloid ergotamine tartrate. It is not recommended for children.

▲/● side-effects/warning: *see* ERGOTAMINE TARTRATE.

Liskonum (*Smith, Kline & French*) is a proprietary drug, available only on prescription, used to treat mania and to prevent manic-depressive illnesses. Produced in the form of

sustained-release tablets, Liskonum is a preparation of lithium carbonate. It is not recommended for children.
▲/✚ side-effects/warning: *see* LITHIUM.

Litarex (*CP Pharmaceuticals*) is a proprietary drug, available only on prescription, used to treat acute mania and to prevent manic-depressive illnesses. Produced in the form of sustained-release tablets, Litarex is a preparation of lithium citrate. It is not recommended for children.
▲/✚ side-effects/warning: *see* LITHIUM.

L

lithium, in the form of lithium carbonate or lithium citrate, is singularly effective in preventing the manic episodes in manic-depressive illness. It may also reduce the frequency and severity of depressive episodes. How it works remains imperfectly understood, but its use is so successful that the side-effects caused by its toxicity are deemed to be justified. Administration is oral in the form of tablets and sustained-release tablets.
▲ side-effects: many long-term patients experience nausea, thirst and excessive urination, gastrointestinal disturbance, weakness and tremor. There may be fluid retention and consequent weight gain. Visual disturbances and increasing gastric problems indicate lithium intoxication.
✚ warning: lithium should not be administered to patients with heart disease, impaired kidney function or imperfect sodium balance in the bloodstream. It should be administered with caution to those who are pregnant or lactating, or who are elderly. Prolonged treatment may cause kidney and thyroid gland dysfunction; prolonged overdosage causes eventual brain disease, convulsions, coma, and finally death. Consequently, blood levels of lithium must be regularly checked for toxicity; thyroid function must be monitored; and there must be adequate intake of fluids and sodium.
Related articles: CAMCOLIT; LISKONUM; LITAREX; PHASAL; PRIADEL.

Lobak (*Sterling Research*) is a proprietary, non-narcotic ANALGESIC, available on prescription only to private patients, used to treat painful muscle spasm. Produced in the form of tablets, Lobak represents a preparation of paracetamol together with the SKELETAL MUSCLE RELAXANT chlormezanone. It is not recommended for children.
▲/✚ side-effects/warning: *see* CHLORMEZANONE; PARACETAMOL.

***local anaesthetic:** *see* ANAESTHETIC.

Lodine (*Ayerst*) is a proprietary, ANTI-INFLAMMATORY, non-narcotic ANALGESIC, available only on prescription, used to treat the pain of rheumatism and of other musculo-skeletal disorders. Produced in the form of capsules, Lodine is a preparation of etodolac. It is not recommended for children.
▲/✚ side-effects/warning: *see* ETODOLAC.

lofepramine is a TRICYCLIC ANTIDEPRESSANT drug of a type that has fewer sedative properties than many others. Used to treat depressive illness, it is thus suited more to the treatment of withdrawn and apathetic patients than to those who are agitated and restless. Administration is oral in the form of tablets.

▲ side-effects: common effects include sedation (affecting driving ability), dry mouth and blurred vision; there may also be difficulty in urinating, sweating and irregular heartbeat, behavioural disturbances, a rash, a state of confusion, and/or a loss of libido. Rarely, there are also blood disorders.

● warning: lofepramine should not be administered to patients who suffer from heart disease or psychosis; it should be administered with caution to patients who suffer from diabetes, epilepsy, liver or thyroid disease, glaucoma or urinary retention; or who are pregnant or lactating. Avoid in patients with severe kidney and liver damage. Withdrawal of treatment must be gradual.
Related article: GAMANIL.

loprazolam is a HYPNOTIC drug, one of the BENZODIAZEPINES, used as a tranquillizer for the short-term treatment of insomnia. Administration is oral in the form of tablets.

▲ side-effects: concentration and speed of reaction are affected. There may also be drowsiness, and unsteadiness; elderly patients may enter a state of confusion. Some patients experience sensitivity reactions. Prolonged use may result in tolerance, and dependence.

● warning: loprazolam should not be administered to patients with acute pulmonary insufficiency (lung disease or shallow breathing) or with myasthenia gravis; it should be administered with caution to those with impaired liver or kidney function, who are pregnant or lactating, or who are elderly and debilitated.
Related article: DORMONOCT.

lorazepam is an ANXIOLYTIC and ANTIDEPRESSANT drug, one of the BENZODIAZEPINES, used to treat mental stress ranging from anxiety to severe panic. It may also be used to treat insomnia, status epilepticus and commonly as a premedication before operations. Administration is oral in the form of tablets, or by injection.

▲ side-effects: concentration and speed of reaction are affected. Drowsiness, unsteadiness, headache, and shallow breathing are all fairly common. Elderly patients may enter a state of confusion. Sensitivity reactions may occur. The drug may enhance the effects of alcohol consumption. This drug may cause dependence.

● warning: lorazepam should be administered with caution to patients with respiratory difficulties, glaucoma, kidney or liver damage, or porphyria and certain psychotic states; who are in the last stages of pregnancy or are lactating; or who are elderly or debilitated. Prolonged use or abrupt withdrawal of the drug should be avoided.
Related articles: ALMAZINE; ATIVAN.

lormetazepam is a HYPNOTIC drug, one of the BENZODIAZEPINES, used in the short-term treatment of insomnia (especially in the elderly because of its short duration of action). Administration is oral in the form of tablets.

▲ side-effects: concentration and speed of reaction are affected. There may also be drowsiness, unsteadiness and dizziness. Some patients experience sensitivity reactions. Prolonged use may result in tolerance, and dependence.

● warning: lormetazepam should

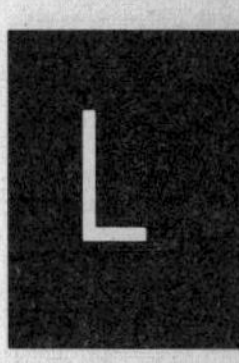

be administered with caution to patients with lung disease or shallow breathing, or impaired liver or kidney function, who are pregnant or lactating, or who are elderly and debilitated.

loxapine is an ANTIPSYCHOTIC drug used as a major TRANQUILLIZER in patients suffering acute and chronic psychotic illness.

▲ side-effects: concentration and speed of thought and movement are affected; the effects of alcohol consumption are enhanced. High doses may cause extrapyramidal movement disorders. Muscle spasms (dystonias) and Parkinsonian-like rigidity, tremor and slow movement may occur. Prolonged use may also cause abnormal compulsive movements of the hands, face and head (tardive dyskinesias). There may be dry mouth and blocked nose, nausea, vomiting, flushing, headache, difficulty in breathing (dyspnoea), constipation and difficulty in urinating, and blurred vision; menstrual disturbances in women or impotence in men may occur, with weight gain; there may be sensitivity reactions. Some patients feel cold and depressed, and tend to suffer from poor sleep patterns. Blood pressure may be low and the heartbeat irregular. Prolonged high dosage may cause opacity in the cornea and lens of the eyes, and a purple pigmentation of the skin. Treatment by intra-muscular injection may be painful.

✚ warning: loxapine should not be administered to patients with certain forms of glaucoma, whose blood-cell formation by the bone-marrow is reduced, or who are taking drugs that depress certain centres of the brain and spinal cord. It should be administered with caution to those with lung disease, cardiovascular disease, epilepsy, parkinsonism, abnormal secretion by the adrenal glands, impaired liver or kidney function, undersecretion of thyroid hormones (hypothyroidism), enlargement of the prostate gland, or any form of acute infection; who are pregnant or lactating; or who are elderly. Prolonged use requires regular checks on eye function and skin pigmentation. Withdrawal of treatment should be gradual. *Related article:* LOXAPAC.

Loxapac (*Lederle*) is a proprietary form of the ANTIPSYCHOTIC drug loxapine. It is available on prescription in the form of capsules (in three strengths).

▲/✚ side-effects/warning: *see* LOXAPINE.

LSD, or lysergide (lysergic acid diethylamide), is a powerful hallucinogenic drug that was occasionally used therapeutically to assist in the treatment of psychological disorders. Although the drug expands awareness and perception, and creates a false world at the same time, there are many toxic side-effects and its use – apart from being illegal – can lead to severely psychotic conditions in which life itself may be at risk. This drug is on the controlled drug list, and is no longer considered by most authorities to be of medical value.

▲ side-effects: usage may cause dizziness and sweating, tingling and dilated pupils, gastrointestinal disturbance and anxiety, tremor and loss of delicate control of the muscles.

✚ warning: LSD should be used only to treat cases for which it is deemed essential. Alteration in the experience of all the senses occurs; psychotic affects are common; confusion and depression may follow.

Ludiomil (*Ciba*) is a proprietary ANTIDEPRESSANT, related to the TRICYCLIC class, available only on prescription, used to treat depressive illness especially in cases where sedation is deemed additionally to be necessary. Produced in the form of tablets (in four strengths), Ludiomil is a preparation of maprotiline hydrochloride. It is not recommended for children.
▲/● side-effects/warning: *see* MAPROTILINE HYDROCHLORIDE.

lysergide is another chemical name for lysergic acid diethylamide, or LSD.
see LSD.

lysuride maleate is a recently introduced ANTIPARKINSONIAN drug that is similar to BROMOCRIPTINE in its actions. It acts by stimulating those dopamine receptors still present in the brain to a suitable extent, and differs from the older form of treatment with levodopa in that the latter is actually converted to DOPAMINE in the brain. It is particularly useful in patients who cannot tolerate levodopa. It is available in the form of tablets.
▲ side-effects: there may be headache, nausea and vomiting, lethargy and drowsiness, hypotension, rashes, psychotic reactions including hallucinations, occasional rashes, constipation and abdominal pain. Care should be taken driving and operating machinery or porphyria.
● warning: should be administered with caution in patients with a psychotic history, or who have had a pituitary tumour. It should not be given to patients with certain severe cardiovascular disorders.
Related article: REVANIL.

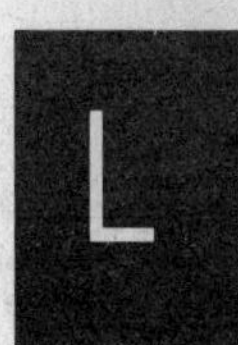

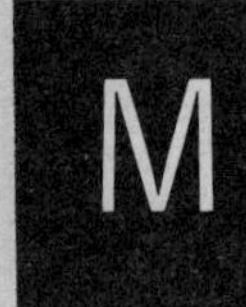

Madopar (*Roche*) is a proprietary preparation of the powerful drug levodopa in combination with the enzyme inhibitor BENSERAZIDE; it is available only on prescription. Madopar is used to treat parkinsonism, but not the parkinsonian symptoms induced by drugs (*see* ANTIPARKINSONIAN). The benserazide prevents too rapid a breakdown of the levodopa (into DOPAMINE), thus allowing more levodopa to reach the brain to make up the deficiency (of dopamine), which is the cause of parkinsonian symptoms. Madopar is produced in the form of capsules (in three strengths), tablets (in two strengths) and as capsules (Madopar CR).

▲/ ● side-effects/warning: *see* LEVODOPA.

***major tranquillizer:** *see* TRANQUILLIZER.

Mantadine (*Du Pont*) is a proprietary preparation of the powerful drug amantadine hydrochloride, available only on prescription, used to treat parkinsonism, but not the parkinsonian symptoms induced by drugs (*see* ANTIPARKINSONIAN). Effective on some patients, but not on others, Mantadine is produced in the form of capsules.

▲/ ● side-effects/warning: *see* AMANTADINE HYDROCHLORIDE.

***MAO inhibitors**, monoamine oxidase inhibitors or MAOI, are one of the major classes of ANTIDEPRESSANTS. Chemically, they are usually hydrazine derivatives. Although they generally enhance confidence in the patient, they are used less often than members of the TRICYCLIC group of antidepressants. MAO inhibitors are also sometimes useful in the treatment of panic disorders. One of the main problems with the use of this class of drug is the risk of serious hypertension (high blood pressure) should a patient accidentally ingest food containing the amine tyramine (present in cheese, meat extracts and many other foods and beverages). Normally tyramine is readily detoxified by the monoamine oxidase enzymes, but if this is inhibited tyramine can cause a massive release of NORADRENALINE and ADRENALINE from nerve and adrenal medullary cells. These in turn cause constriction of blood vessels and so raising blood pressure.

maprotiline hydrochloride is an ANTIDEPRESSANT drug, related to the TRICYCLIC CLASS, used to treat depressive illness, particularly in cases where some degree of sedation is called for. Administration is oral in the form of tablets, or by intramuscular or intravenous injection.

▲ side-effects: common effects include sedation (affecting driving ability), dry mouth, rashes and blurred vision; there may also be difficulty in urinating, sweating and irregular heartbeat, behavioural disturbances, a state of confusion, and/or a loss of libido. At higher doses rashes commonly occur and there may be convulsions. Rarely, there are also blood disorders.

● warning: maprotiline hydrochloride should not be administered to patients who suffer from heart disease or psychosis; it should be administered with caution to patients who suffer from diabetes, epilepsy, liver or thyroid disease, glaucoma or urinary retention; or who are pregnant or lactating.

Withdrawal of treatment must be gradual.
Related article: LUDIOMIL.

Marplan (*Roche*) is a proprietary ANTIDEPRESSANT drug of the MAO INHIBITOR class, available only on prescription, used to treat depressive illness. Produced in the form of tablets, Marplan is a preparation of the potentially dangerous drug isocarboxazid (which requires a careful dietary regimen to accompany treatment). It is not suitable for children.
▲/ ✚ side-effects/warning: *see* ISOCARBOXAZID.

Marzine RF (*Wellcome*) is a proprietary form of the ANTIHISTAMINE cinnarizine used as an ANTI-EMETIC and available without prescription to prevent travel sickness.
▲/ ✚ side-effects/warning: *see* CINNARIZINE.

Maxolon (*Beecham*) is a proprietary ANTINAUSEANT, used to treat severe indigestion, flatulence, peptic, gastric or duodenal ulcer, hiatus hernia or gallstones. Available only on prescription, Maxolon's primary constituent – metoclopramide hydrochloride – works by encouraging the flow of absorbable nutrients in food in the stomach down into the intestines. It is produced in the form of tablets, in liquid form (under the name Maxolon Paediatric Liquid), as a syrup (under the name Maxolon Syrup) and in ampoules for injection (under the names Maxolon Injection and Maxolon High Dose).
▲/ ✚ side-effects/warning: *see* METOCLOPRAMIDE.

mazindol is a drug used to aid slimming regimes because it acts as an APPETITE SUPPRESSANT. It has STIMULANT properties, however, and there is a risk of dependence (addiction). Administration is oral in the form of tablets. The drug should be used only in cases where there is genuine medical need for weight loss, and is not recommended for children.
▲ side-effects: there may be agitation, insomnia and restlessness, and a increased heart rate; headache and dizziness may occur; there may also be gastrointestinal disturbances. In predisposed patients there may be manic episodes.
✚ warning: mazindol is merely an aid to a slimming regime, not a treatment for obesity. Its use should be short-term only. Prolonged treatment may result in dependence (addiction). It should not be administered to patients with glaucoma or from disorders of the thyroid gland, to those with epilepsy, diabetes, heart disease or peptic ulcer, or who are unstable psychologically.
Related article: TERONAC.

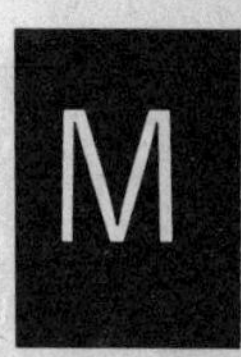

meclozine is an ANTIHISTAMINE used primarily as an ANTI-EMETIC in the treatment or prevention of motion sickness and vomiting. Administration (as meclozine hydrochloride, generally with a form of vitamin B) is oral in the form of tablets.
▲ side-effects: concentration and speed of thought and movement may be affected. There is commonly dry mouth and drowsiness; there may also be headache, blurred vision and gastrointestinal disturbances.
✚ warning: meclazine should be administered with caution to patients with epilepsy, liver disease, glaucoma or enlargement of the prostate gland. Drowsiness may be

increased by alcohol consumption.
Related article: SEA-LEGS.

medazepam is an ANXIOLYTIC drug, one of the BENZODIAZEPINES, used primarily for the short-term treatment of anxiety, and less commonly, insomnia. It may also be used to relieve acute alcohol withdrawal symptoms. It also has the properties of a SKELETAL MUSCLE RELAXANT, and may also be administered to relieve conditions of skeletal muscle spasticity. Administration is oral in the form of capsules.

▲ side-effects: concentration and speed of reaction are affected. Drowsiness, unsteadiness, headache, and shallow breathing are all fairly common. Elderly patients may enter a state of confusion. Sensitivity reactions may occur.

⬢ warning: medazepam should be administered with caution to patients with respiratory difficulties, glaucoma, or kidney or liver disease; who are in the last stages of pregnancy or are lactating; or who are elderly or debilitated. Dependence readily occurs and abrupt withdrawal of the drug should be avoided.
Related article: NOBRIUM.

Medihaler-Ergotamine (*Riker*) is a proprietary anti-migraine treatment, available only on prescription, used in the form of an inhalant to treat migraine and recurrent vascular headache. Produced in a metered-dosage aerosol, Medihaler-Ergotamine is a preparation of the vegetable alkaloid ergotamine tartrate.

▲/⬢ side-effects/warning: *see* ERGOTAMINE TARTRATE.

Medised (*Martindale/Panpharma*) is a proprietary, non-prescription, compound non-narcotic ANALGESIC, which is not available from the National Health Service. Used to treat pain, especially that associated with fever and respiratory congestion. Medised is produced in the form of a suspension (which is not recommended for children aged under 3 months). Medised is a combination of the analgesic paracetamol and the ANTIHISTAMINE promethazine hydrochloride.

▲/⬢ side-effects/warning: *see* PARACETAMOL; PROMETHAZINE HYDROCHLORIDE.

Medocodene (*Medo*) is a proprietary, non-prescription compound ANALGESIC, which is not available from the National Health Service. Used to treat pain anywhere in the body, and produced in the form of tablets, Medocodene is a combination of the analgesic paracetamol and the OPIATE analgesic codeine phosphate (a combination itself known as co-codamol). It is not recommended for children aged under 6 years.

▲/⬢ side-effects/warning: *see* CODEINE PHOSPHATE; PARACETAMOL.

mefenamic acid is a non-steroidal, ANTI-INFLAMMATORY, non-narcotic ANALGESIC. It is primarily used to treat mild to moderate pain in rheumatic disease and other musculo-skeletal disorders, although it may also be used either to reduce high body temperature (especially in children) or to lessen the pain of menstrual problems.

▲ side-effects: there may be drowsiness and dizziness; some patients experience nausea; gastrointestinal disturbances may eventually result in ulceration and rashes. Treatment should be withdrawn if diarrhoea, jaundice, anaemia or sensitivity reactions such as asthma-like symptoms occur.

● warning: mefenamic acid should not be administered to patients with inflammations in the intestines, peptic ulcers, or impaired liver or kidney function; or who are pregnant. It should be administered with caution to those with any allergic condition (including asthma). Prolonged treatment requires regular blood counts.
Related article: PONSTAN.

Melleril (*Sandoz*) is a proprietary form of the ANTIPSYCHOTIC drug thioridazine. Available only on prescription, it is used to treat and tranquillize psychosis (such as schizophrenia) in which it is particularly suitable for treating manic forms of behavioural disturbance. It may also be used to treat anxiety in the short term. Melleril is produced in the form of tablets (in four strengths), as a suspension (in two strengths) and as a syrup for dilution (the potency of the syrup once dilute is retained for 14 days).

▲/● side-effects/warning: *see* THIORIDAZINE.

meprobamate is a minor TRANQUILLIZER and ANXIOLYTIC used in the short-term treatment of anxiety. It may also be used to assist in the treatment of minor forms of neurosis. Prolonged treatment, however, may lead to tolerance and dependence (addiction), and this drug is dangerous in overdose. Administration is oral in the form of tablets.

▲ side-effects: concentration and speed of thought and movement are affected; the degree of sedation may be marked. There may also be low blood pressure (hypotension), debility, gastrointestinal disturbances, headache, blurred vision and rashes. The effect of alcohol consumption may be enhanced.

● warning: meprobamate should not be administered to patients with porphyria, or who are lactating. It should be administered with caution to those with respiratory difficulties, glaucoma, epilepsy, or impaired liver or kidney function, who are in the last stages of pregnancy, or who are elderly or debilitated. Withdrawal of treatment must be gradual (abrupt withdrawal may cause convulsions).
Related articles: EQUAGESIC; EQUANIL.

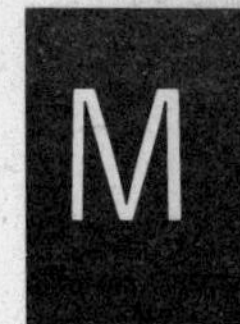

meptazinol is a powerful synthetic NARCOTIC ANALGESIC, an OPIATE that is used to treat moderate to severe pain, including pain in childbirth or following surgery. The onset of its effect is said to take place within 15 minutes of injection, and the duration is said to be between 2 and 7 hours; however, there are some post-operative side-effects. Administration is also oral in the form of tablets.

▲ side-effects: nausea, vomiting, dizziness, sweating and drowsiness are fairly common. However, unlike most drugs of its type, meptazinol is said not to cause shallow breathing.

● warning: meptazinol should not be administered to patients with head injury or raised intracranial pressure; it should be administered with caution to those with impaired kidney or liver function, asthma, depressed respiration, insufficient secretion of thyroid hormones (hypothyroidism) or low blood pressure (hypotension), or who are pregnant or lactating. Dosage should be decreased for the elderly or debilitated.
Related article: MEPTID.

Meptid (*Wyeth*) is a proprietary NARCOTIC ANALGESIC, available only on prescription, used to treat moderate to severe pain, particularly during or following surgical procedures (including childbirth). Produced in the form of tablets and in ampoules for injection, Meptid is a preparation of the OPIATE meptazinol, and is not recommended for children.
▲/✚ side-effects/warning: *see* MEPTAZINOL.

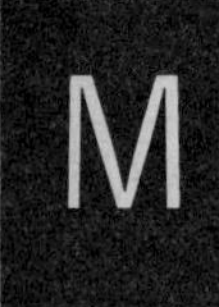

mepyramine is an ANTIHISTAMINE used to treat the symptoms of allergic conditions such as hay fever and urticaria, and – as an ANTI-EMETIC – to treat or prevent nausea and vomiting, especially in connection with motion sickness or the vertigo caused by infection of the middle or inner ear. Administration (as mepyramine maleate) is oral in the form of tablets.
▲ side-effects: sedation may affect patients' capacity for speed of thought and movement; there may be headache and/or weight gain, dry mouth, gastrointestinal disturbances and visual problems.
✚ warning: mepyramine should not be administered to patients with glaucoma, urinary retention, intestinal obstruction, enlargement of the prostate gland, or peptic ulcer, or who are pregnant; it should be administered with caution to those with epilepsy or liver disease.

methadone is a powerful and long-acting narcotic ANALGESIC used both to relieve severe pain and – like several narcotic analgesics – to suppress coughs. One of its principal uses is in the treatment of heroin addicts. Prolonged use of methadone can, however, also lead to dependence (addiction). Administration (in the form of methadone hydrochloride) is oral in the form of tablets, as a linctus, or by injection.
▲ side-effects: there is commonly constipation, drowsiness and dizziness. High dosage may result in respiratory depression.
✚ warning: methadone should not be administered to patients with liver disease, raised intracranial pressure, or head injury. It should be administered with caution to those with asthma, low blood pressure (hypotension), underactivity of the thyroid gland (hypothyroidism) or impaired liver or kidney function; who are pregnant or lactating; who are taking monoamine oxidase inhibitors; or have a history of drug abuse. Its effect is cumulative. Dosage should be reduced for elderly or debilitated patients.
Related article: PHYSEPTONE.

methionine is an antidote to poisoning by the analgesic paracetamol (which has the greatest toxic effect on the liver). Administration is oral in the form of tablets; dosage depends on the results of blood counts every 4 hours.

methixene hydrochloride is a powerful ANTIPARKINSONIAN drug, used to relieve some of the symptoms of parkinsonism, specifically the tremor of the hands, the overall rigidity of the posture, and the tendency to produce an excess of saliva, but not tardive dyskinesia. (The drug also has the capacity to treat these conditions in some cases where they are produced by drugs.) It is thought to work by compensating for the lack of the neurotransmitter DOPAMINE in the brain, which is the major cause of such parkinsonian symptoms. Administration – which may be in parallel with the administration of LEVODOPA – is oral in the form of tablets.

▲ side-effects: there may be dry mouth, dizziness and blurred vision, and/or gastrointestinal disturbances. Some patients experience sensitivity reactions and anxiety. Rarely, and in susceptible patients, there may be confusion, agitation and psychological disturbance (at which point treatment must be withdrawn).

● warning: methixene hydrochloride should not be administered to patients with not merely tremor but with distinct involuntary movements; it should be administered with caution to those with impaired kidney or liver function, cardiovascular disease, glaucoma, or urinary retention. Withdrawal of treatment must be gradual.
Related article: TREMONIL.

methohexitone sodium is a general ANAESTHETIC used for both the induction and the maintenance of general anaesthesia in surgical operations; administration is intravenous (generally in 1% solution). It is less irritant to tissues than some other anaesthetics, and recovery afterwards is quick, but the induction of anaesthesia is not particularly smooth.

▲ side-effects: induction may cause hiccups and involuntary movements. The patient may feel pain on the initial injection.

● warning: maintenance of anaesthesia is usually in combination with other anaesthetics. Induction may take up to 60 seconds.
Related article: BRIETAL SODIUM.

methotrimeprazine is an ANTIPSYCHOTIC drug of the phenothiazine class, similar in its effects to chlorpromazine. It may be used in the treatment of psychoses, but its particular use is for its TRANQUILLIZER and ANTI-EMETIC actions in patients who are dying. Administration is oral in the form of tablets or by injection.

▲ side-effects: concentration and speed of thought and movement are affected; the effects of alcohol may be enhanced. There may be dry mouth and blocked nose, constipation and difficulty in urinating, and blurred vision; menstrual disturbances in women or impotence in men may occur, with weight gain; there may be sensitivity reactions. Some patients feel cold and depressed, and tend to suffer from poor sleep patterns. Blood pressure may be low and the heartbeat irregular. Prolonged high dosage may cause extrapyramidal motor disorders, opacity in the cornea and lens of the eyes, and a purple pigmentation of the skin. Treatment by intramuscular injection may be painful.

● warning: methotrimeprazine should not be administered to patients with certain forms of glaucoma, whose blood-cell formation by the bone-marrow is reduced, or who are taking drugs that depress certain centres of the brain and spinal cord. It should be administered with caution to those with lung disease, cardiovascular disease, epilepsy, parkinsonism, abnormal secretion by the adrenal glands, impaired liver or kidney function, undersecretion of thyroid hormones (hypothyroidism),

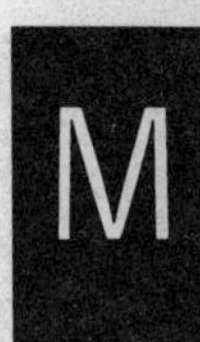

enlargement of the prostate gland or any form of acute infection; who are pregnant or lactating; or who are elderly. Prolonged use requires regular physical checks. Withdrawal of treatment should be gradual. *Related article:* NOZINAN.

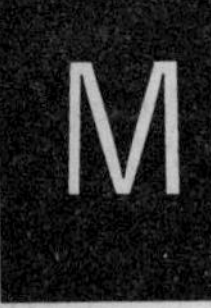

methylphenobarbitone is a drug used to treat grand mal (tonic-clonic) and focal (partial) seizures of epilepsy. Administered orally in the form of tablets, it is converted in the liver to the powerful SEDATIVE and ANTICONVULSANT BARBITURATE phenobarbitone, with which it shares action and effects.

▲/● side-effects/warning: *see see* PHENOBARBITONE.

methysergide is a potentially dangerous drug used, generally under strict medical supervision in a hospital, to prevent severe recurrent migraine and similar headaches in patients for whom other forms of treatment have failed. Administration is oral in the form of tablets.

▲ side-effects: there is initial nausea, drowsiness and dizziness; there may also be fluid retention and consequent weight gain, spasm of the arteries, insomnia, cramps, loss of hair, numbness of the fingers and toes, increased heart rate and even psychological changes.

● warning: methysergide should not be administered to patients with heart, lung, liver or kidney disease, or who suffer from collagen disorders, or who are pregnant or lactating. It should be administered with caution to those with peptic ulcer. Withdrawal of treatment should be gradual, although no course of treatment should last for more than 6 months at a time.

metoclopramide is an effective ANTI-EMETIC and ANTINAUSEANT drug, which also has MOTILITY STIMULANT properties, and may be used to prevent vomiting caused by gastrointestinal disorders or by chemotherapy or radiotherapy in the treatment of cancer. It works both by direct action on the vomiting centre of the brain and by actions within the intestinal walls to increase the rate of emptying of the stomach and increase the passage of food products along the intestine. In this respect some newer drugs such as CISAPRIDE are effective but with fewer side-effects. Although as an anti-emetic metoclopramide has fewer side-effects than some others (such as the phenothiazine derivatives), newer agents such as ONDANSETRON may now prove more beneficial. Administration (as metoclopramide hydrochloride) is oral in the form of tablets and syrups, or by injection.

▲ side-effects: side-effects are relatively uncommon, especially in male patients. There may, however, be mild neuromuscular symptoms, drowsiness, restlessness and diarrhoea.

● warning: metoclopramide should not be administered to patients who have had gastrointestinal surgery within the previous 4 days; it should be administered with caution to those with impaired kidney function, or who are children, pregnant, lactating or elderly. Dosage should begin low and gradually increase. The effects of the drug may mask underlying disorders. *Related articles:* GASTROBID CONTINUS; GASTROMAX; MAXOLON; METOX; METRAMID; PARMID; PRIMPERAN.

metoprolol is a BETA-BLOCKER used to prevent recurrent attacks of migraine. Administration (as metoprolol tartrate) is oral in the form of tablets and sustained-release tablets, or by injection.

▲ side-effects: there may be some gastrointestinal or slight respiratory disturbance following oral administration. Some patients experience sensitivity reactions.

● warning: as a hypertensive drug, metoprolol tartrate should not be administered to patients with heart disease or asthmatic symptoms; it should be administered with caution to those with impaired kidney function, or who are nearing the end of pregnancy or lactating. Withdrawal of treatment should be gradual. *Related article:* BETALOC.

Metox (*Steinhard*) is a proprietary preparation of the ANTI-EMETIC drug metoclopramide hydrochloride, available only on prescription, used to relieve symptoms of nausea and vomiting caused by gastrointestinal disorders, or by chemotherapy or radiotherapy in the treatment of cancer. It is produced in the form of tablets.

▲/● side-effects/warning: *see* METOCLOPRAMIDE.

Metramid (*Nicholas*) is a proprietary preparation of the ANTI-EMETIC drug metoclopramide hydrochloride, available only on prescription, used to relieve symptoms of nausea and vomiting caused by gastrointestinal disorders, or by chemotherapy or radiotherapy in the treatment of cancer. It is produced in the form of tablets, and is not recommended for children aged under 15 years.

▲/● side-effects/warning: *see* METOCLOPRAMIDE.

mianserin is an ANTIDEPRESSANT drug used to treat depressive illness, especially in cases in which a degree of sedation may be useful. Administration is oral in the form of tablets.

▲ side-effects: common effects include sedation (affecting driving ability), dry mouth and blurred vision; there may also be difficulty in urinating, sweating and irregular heartbeat, behavioural disturbances, a rash, a state of confusion, and/or a loss of libido. Rarely, there are also blood disorders.

● warning: mianserin should not be administered to patients who suffer from heart disease or psychosis; it should be administered with caution to patients who suffer from diabetes, epilepsy, liver or thyroid disease, glaucoma or urinary retention; or who are pregnant or lactating. Withdrawal of treatment must be gradual. *Related article:* LUDIOMIL; NORVAL.

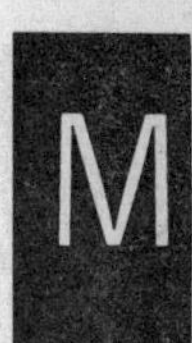

Microfen (*Chatfield Laboratories*) is a proprietary, non-narcotic, ANALGESIC containing ibuprofen, which also has ANTI-INFLAMMATORY properties (NSAID). It is available without prescription as tablets (in three strengths).

▲/● side-effects/warning: *see* IBUPROFEN.

midazolam is an ANXIOLYTIC drug, one of the BENZODIAZEPINES, used primarily to provide sedation for minor surgery such as dental operations or as a premedication prior to surgical procedures and, because it also has some SKELETAL MUSCLE RELAXANT properties, to treat some forms of spasm. Prolonged use results in tolerance and may lead to dependence (addiction), especially in patients

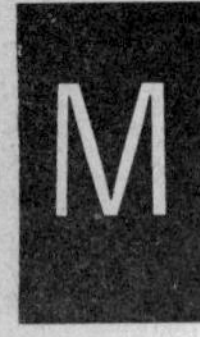

with a history of drug (including alcohol) abuse. Administration is by injection.

▲ side-effects: there may be drowsiness, unsteadiness, headache, and shallow breathing; hypersensitivity reactions may occur.

● warning: concentration and speed of thought and movement are often affected. Midazolam should be administered with caution to patients with respiratory difficulties (it sometimes causes a sharp fall in blood pressure), glaucoma, or kidney or liver disease; who are in especially the last stages of pregnancy; or who are elderly or debilitated. Abrupt withdrawal of treatment should be avoided. *Related articles:* DIAZEPAM; HYPNOVEL.

Midrid (*Carnrick*) is a proprietary compound non-narcotic ANALGESIC, available only on prescription, used to treat migraine and other headaches caused by tension. Produced in the form of capsules, Midrid is a preparation of the SYMPATHOMIMETIC isometheptene mucate, the SEDATIVE dichloralphenazone and the analgesic paracetamol; it is not recommended for prescription to children.

▲/● side-effects/warning: *see* ISOMETHEPTENE MUCATE; PARACETAMOL.

Migraleve (*International Labs*) is a proprietary, non-prescription compound ANALGESIC and ANTIHISTAMINE, used to treat migraine. Produced in the form of tablets, Migraleve is a preparation of the antihistamine buclizine hydrochloride, the analgesic paracetamol and the OPIATE codeine phosphate; tablets without buclizine hydrochloride are also available separately or in a duo-pack. These preparations are not recommended for children aged under 10 years. They should never be used prophylactically.

▲/● side-effects/warning: *see* CODEINE PHOSPHATE; PARACETAMOL.

Migravess (*Bayer*) is a proprietary, compound non-narcotic ANALGESIC, available only on prescription, used to treat migraine. Produced in the form of tablets (in two strengths, the stronger under the name Migravess Forte), Migravess is a preparation of the analgesic aspirin together with the ANTI-EMETIC metoclopramide hydrochloride. It is not recommended for children aged under 10 years.

▲/● side-effects/warning: *see* ASPIRIN; METOCLOPRAMIDE.

Migril (*Wellcome*) is a proprietary, compound non-narcotic ANALGESIC, available only on prescription, used to treat migraine and some other vascular headaches. Produced in the form of tablets, Migril is a preparation of the vegetable alkaloid ergotamine tartrate, the ANTIHISTAMINE cyclizine hydrochloride and the mild STIMULANT caffeine hydrate. It is not recommended for children.

▲/● side-effects/warning: *see* CYCLIZINE; ERGOTAMINE TARTRATE.

Min-I-Jet Morphine Sulphate (*IMS*) is a proprietary form of the narcotic ANALGESIC morphine, which is on the controlled drugs list. It is available on prescription only, as an injection.

▲/● side-effects/warning: *see* MORPHINE.

***minor tranquillizer:** *see* TRANQUILLIZER; ANXIOLYTIC.

Mobiflex (*Roche*) is a proprietary form of the non-steroidal, ANTI-INFLAMMATORY, non-narcotic

ANALGESIC drug tenoxicam. It is available on prescription as tablets to treat the pain and inflammation associated with osteoarthritis and rheumatoid arthritis.
▲/ ♣ side-effects/warning: *see* TENOXICAM.

Mobilan (*Galen*) is a proprietary, ANTI-INFLAMMATORY, non-narcotic ANALGESIC, available only on prescription, used to treat the pain of rheumatic and other musculo-skeletal disorders (including gout, bursitis and tendonitis). Produced in the form of capsules (in two strengths), Mobilan is a preparation of indomethacin.
▲/ ♣ side-effects/warning: *see* INDOMETHACIN.

Modecate (*Squibb*) is a proprietary ANTIPSYCHOTIC drug, available only on prescription, used in the long-term maintenance of tranquillization for patients suffering from psychoses (including schizophrenia). Produced in ampoules for injection (in two strengths, the stronger under the trade name Modecate Concentrate), Modecate is a preparation of fluphenazine decanoate. It is not recommended for children.
▲/ ♣ side-effects/warning: *see* FLUPHENAZINE.

Moditen (*Squibb*) is a proprietary ANTIPSYCHOTIC drug, available only on prescription, used in the long-term maintenance, as a major TRANQUILLIZER, for patients suffering from psychoses (including schizophrenia) and patients with behavioural disturbances. It may also be used in the short term to treat severe anxiety. Produced in the form of tablets (in three strengths), Moditen is a preparation of fluphenazine hydrochloride. Ampoules for depot injection are also available (under the name Moditen Enanthate) containing fluphenazine enanthate. Neither of these preparations is recommended for children.
▲/ ♣ side-effects/warning: *see* FLUPHENAZINE.

Mogadon (*Roche*) is a proprietary HYPNOTIC, available on prescription only to private patients, used to treat insomnia in cases where some degree of daytime sedation is acceptable. Produced in the form of tablets and as capsules, Mogadon is a preparation of the long-acting BENZODIAZEPINE nitrazepam, and is not recommended for children.
▲/ ♣ side-effects/warning: *see* NITRAZEPAM.

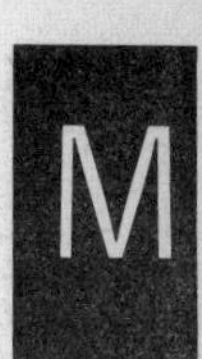

Molipaxin (*Roussel*) is a proprietary ANTIDEPRESSANT, available only on prescription, used to treat depressive illness (especially in cases where there is anxiety). It causes sedation. Produced in the form of capsules (in two strengths) and as a sugar-free liquid, Molipaxin is a preparation of the drug trazodone hydrochloride; it is not recommended for children.
▲/ ♣ side-effects/warning: *see* TRAZODONE HYDROCHLORIDE.

***monoamine oxidase inhibitor:** *see* MAO INHIBITOR.

morphine is a powerful NARCOTIC ANALGESIC, which is the principal alkaloid of opium. It is widely used to treat severe pain and to soothe the associated stress and anxiety; it may be used in treating shock (with care since it lowers blood pressure), in suppressing coughs (an ANTITUSSIVE – although it may cause nausea and vomiting), and in reducing peristalsis (the muscular waves that urge material along the intestines) as a constituent in some antidiarrhoeal mixtures. It

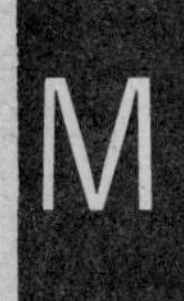

is also sometimes used as a premedication prior to surgery, or to supplement anaesthesia during an operation. Tolerance occurs extremely readily; dependence (addiction) may follow. Administration is oral, by injection, and as rectal suppositories; given by injection, morphine is more active. Proprietary preparations that contain morphine (in the form of morphine, morphine tartrate, morphine hydrochloride or morphine sulphate) are all on the controlled drugs list.

▲ side-effects: there may be nausea and vomiting, loss of appetite and constipation. There is generally a degree of sedation, and euphoria which may lead to a state of mental detachment or confusion. There may be difficulty in urination, dry mouth, vertigo, flushing, miosis (excessive contraction of the pupil), palpitations, postural hypotension, hypothermia, urticaria and pruritus (itching).

● warning: morphine should not be administered to patients with depressed breathing (the drug may itself cause a degree of respiratory depression), or who have raised intracranial pressure or head injury. It should be administered with caution to those with low blood pressure (hypotension), impaired liver or kidney function, asthma, hypotension, or underactivity of the thyroid gland (hypothyroidism); or who are pregnant or lactating. Dosage should be reduced for the elderly or debilitated. Treatment by injection may cause pain and tissue damage at the site of the injection. Prolonged treatment should be avoided.

Related articles: CYCLIMORPH; MIN-I-JET MORPHINE SULPHATE; MST CONTINUS; NEPENTHE; ORAMORPH; SEVREDOL.

***motility stimulants** are a class of drugs, newly recognised, that stimulate stomach emptying and the rate of passage of food products along the small intestine, and may also enhance closure of the oesphageal sphincter thereby reducing reflux passage of stomach contents up into the oesophagus. Under the condition that they are used carefully, such drugs are of benefit because they have ANTI-NAUSEANT and ANTI-EMETIC properties. Older drugs of this class, such as METOCLOPRIMIDE, had DOPAMINE receptor antagonist properties, so they had a wide variety of undesirable effects on the brain. Some recently introduced agents such as cisapride do not have this action, and are thought to work by acting at receptors for 5-HT (serotonin) to cause release of the neurotransmitter acetylcholine from nerves within the gut wall.

Motilium (*Janssen*) is a proprietary preparation of the ANTINAUSEANT and ANTI-EMETIC drug domperidone, available only on prescription. It is thought to work by inhibiting the action of the neurotransmitter DOPAMINE on the vomiting centre of the brain, and may be used to treat nausea and vomiting in gastrointestinal disorders, or during treatment with cytotoxic drugs or radiotherapy. It is produced in the form of tablets, as a sugar-free suspension and as anal suppositories.

▲/● side-effects/warning: *see* DOMPERIDONE.

Motipress (*Squibb*) is a proprietary mixed ANTIDEPRESSANT-ANTIPSYCHOTIC compound, available only on prescription,

used to treat depressive illness and associated anxiety. Produced in the form of tablets, Motipress is a preparation of the antipsychotic drug fluphenazine hydrochloride and the antidepressant nortriptyline hydrochloride in the ratio 1:20. It is not recommended for children.
▲/✚ side-effects/warning: *see* FLUPHENAZINE; NORTRIPTYLINE.

Motival (*Squibb*) is a proprietary mixed ANTIDEPRESSANT-ANTIPSYCHOTIC compound, available only on prescription, used to treat depressive illness and associated anxiety. Produced in the form of tablets, Motival is a preparation of the antipsychotic drug fluphenazine hydrochloride and the antidepressant nortriptyline hydrochloride in the ratio 50:1. It is not recommended for children.
▲/✚ side-effects/warning: *see* FLUPHENAZINE; NORTRIPTYLINE.

Motrin (*Upjohn*) is a proprietary, ANTI-INFLAMMATORY, non-narcotic ANALGESIC, available only on prescription, used to treat the pain of rheumatic and other musculo-skeletal disorders. Produced in the form of tablets (in four strengths), Motrin is a preparation of ibuprofen.
▲/✚ side-effects/warning: *see* IBUPROFEN.

MST Continus (*Napp*) is a proprietary NARCOTIC ANALGESIC, which is on the controlled drugs list. It is used primarily to relieve pain following surgery, or the pain experienced during the final stages of terminal malignant disease. Produced in the form of sustained-release tablets (in four strengths), MST Continus is a preparation of the OPIATE and narcotic morphine sulphate; it is not recommended for children.
▲/✚ side-effects/warning: *see* MORPHINE.

Mygdalon (*DDSA Pharmaceuticals*) is a proprietary ANTINAUSEANT, available only on prescription, used to treat nausea and vomiting especially when associated with gastrointestinal disorders, during radiotherapy, or accompanying treatment with cytotoxic drugs. Produced in the form of tablets, Mygdalon is a preparation of metoclopramide hydrochloride.
▲/✚ side-effects/warning: *see* METOCLOPRAMIDE.

Mysoline (*ICI*) is a proprietary ANTICONVULSANT, available only on prescription, used to treat and prevent epileptic attacks, especially grand mal (tonic-clonic) and partial (focal) seizures (but not petit mal epilepsy). Produced in the form of tablets and an oral suspension, Mysoline is a preparation of primidone.
▲/✚ side-effects/warning: *see* PRIMIDONE.

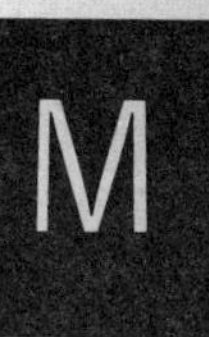

nabilone is a synthetic cannabinoid (a drug derived from CANNABIS) used as an ANTI-EMETIC to relieve some of the toxic side-effects, particularly the nausea and vomiting, associated with chemotherapy in the treatment of cancer. However, it too has significant side-effects. Administration is oral in the form of capsules.

▲ side-effects: drowsiness, dry mouth and decreased appetite are common; there may also be an increase in the heart rate, dizziness on rising from a sitting or lying position (indicating low blood pressure), and abdominal cramps. Some patients experience psychological effects such as euphoria, confusion, depression, hallucinations and general disorientation. There may be headache, blurred vision and tremors.

● warning: nabilone should be administered with caution to patients with severely impaired liver function or unstable personality. Concentration and speed of reaction is affected, and the effects of alcohol may be increased.
Related article: CESAMET.

nabumetone is a non-steroidal, ANTI-INFLAMMATORY, non-narcotic ANALGESIC drug used to treat pain and inflammation in rheumatoid arthritis and osteoarthritis.

▲ side-effects: administration with or following meals reduces the risk of gastrointestinal disturbance and nausea. There may be headache, dizziness and ringing in the ears (tinnitus), and some patients experience sensitivity reactions or blood disorders. Occasionally, there is fluid retention.

● warning: nabumetone should be administered with caution to patients with impaired liver or kidney function, gastric ulcers, or severe allergies (including asthma), or who are pregnant.
Related article: RELIFEX.

nadolol is a BETA-BLOCKER used as an ANTIMIGRAINE treatment to reduce the frequency of attacks. Administration is oral in the form of tablets.

▲ side-effects: the heartbeat may slow more than intended; there may be some gastrointestinal or respiratory disturbance. Fingers and toes may turn cold.

● warning: nadolol should not be administered to patients who suffer from heart disease or asthma, and should be administered with caution to those who are nearing the end of pregnancy or who are lactating. Withdrawal of treatment should be gradual.
Related article: CORGARD.

nalbuphine hydrochloride is a NARCOTIC ANALGESIC that is very similar to morphine (although it has fewer side-effects and possibly less addictive potential). Like morphine, it is used primarily to relieve moderate to severe pain, especially during or after surgery. Administration is by injection.

▲ side-effects: shallow breathing, urinary retention, constipation, and nausea are all common; tolerance and dependence (addiction) are possible. There may also be drowsiness and pain at the site of injection (where there may also be tissue damage).

● warning: nalbuphine should not be administered to patients who suffer from head injury or raised intracranial pressure; it should be administered with caution to those with impaired kidney or liver function, asthma, depressed respiration, insufficient secretion of thyroid hormones (hypothyroidism) or low blood pressure (hypotension), or who are

pregnant or lactating. Dosage should be reduced for the elderly or debilitated.
Related article: NUBAIN.

Nalorex (*Du Pont*) is an antagonist of NARCOTIC ANALGESIC drugs, chemically an OPIATE, and is used in detoxification therapy for formerly opiate-dpendent individuals to help prevent relapse. It is a proprietary form of naltrexone hydrochloride available only on prescription, and is a preparation in the form of tablets.
▲/⬢ side-effects/warning: *see* NALTREXONE HYDROCHLORIDE.

naloxone is a powerful OPIATE antagonist drug used primarily (in the form of naloxone hydrochloride) as an antidote to an overdose of narcotic ANALGESICS. Quick but short-acting, it effectively reverses the respiratory depression, coma and convulsions that follow over-dosage of opiates. Administration is by intramuscular or intravenous injection, and may be repeated at intervals of 2 minutes until there is some response. Also used at the end of operations to reverse respiratory depression caused by narcotic analgesics.
⬢ warning: naloxone should not be administered to patients who are physically dependent on narcotics.
Related article: NARCAN.

naltrexone hydrochloride is an antagonist of NARCOTIC ANALGESIC drugs, chemically an OPIATE, and is used in detoxification therapy for formerly opiate-dependent individuals to help prevent relapse. Since it is an antagonist of dependence-forming opiates (such as heroin), it will precipitate withdrawal symptoms in those already taking opiates. During naltrexone treatment, the euphoric effects of habit-forming opiates are blocked, so helping prevent re-addiction in former addicts. Naltrexone should be used in specialist clinics only. (For overdose with opiates the related drug NALOXONE is normally used). It is available only on prescription in the form of tablets.
▲ side-effects: in withdrawal of opiate-dependent patients there may be nausea, vomiting, abdominal pain, anxiety, nervousness, difficulty in sleeping, headache, and pain in joints and muscles. There may also be diarrhoea or constipation, sweating, dizziness, chills, irritability, rash, lethargy, and decreased sexual potency. There have been reports of liver and blood abnormalities.
⬢ warning: kidney and liver impairment (function tests before and during treatment are advisable). Test for opiate dependence with naloxone, avoid giving to patients currently dependent on opiates, or those with acute hepatic or renal failure.
Related article: NALOREX.

Naprosyn (*Syntex*) is a proprietary, non-steroidal, ANTI-INFLAMMATORY (NSAID), non-narcotic ANALGESIC, available only on prescription, used to relieve pain – particularly rheumatic and arthritic pain, and that of acute gout – and to treat other musculo-skeletal disorders. Produced in the form of tablets (in two strengths), as a suspension (the potency of the suspension once dilute is retained for 14 days), and as anal suppositories, Naprosyn is a preparation of naproxen. In the form of tablets or suspension it is not recommended for children aged under 5 years; the suppositories

are not suitable for children.
▲/ ✚ side-effects/warning: *see* NAPROXEN.

naproxen is a non-steroidal, ANTI-INFLAMMATORY (NSAID), non-narcotic ANALGESIC used to relieve pain – particularly rheumatic and arthritic pain, and that of acute gout – and to treat other musculo-skeletal disorders. It is also effective in relieving the pain of menstrual disorders, in treating migraine, and in reducing high body temperature. Administration (in the form of naproxen or naproxen sodium) is oral in the form of tablets or as a dilute suspension, or by anal suppositories.

▲ side-effects: include gastrointestinal disturbance with nausea; patients may be advised to take the drug with food or milk. Some patients experience sensitivity reactions or fluid retention in the tissues (oedema).

✚ warning: naproxen should be administered with caution to patients with allergic disorders (such as asthma), impaired liver or kidney function, or gastric ulcers, or who are pregnant.
Related articles: ARTHROXEN; LARAFLEX; NAPROSYN; NYCOPREN; SYNFLEX; VALROX.

Narcan (*Du Pont*) is a proprietary drug, available only on prescription, that is most often used to treat the symptoms of acute overdosage of OPIATES such as morphine. Produced in ampoules for injection, Narcan is a preparation of naloxone hydrochloride. A weaker form is available (under the name Narcan Neonatal) for the treatment of respiratory depression in babies born to mothers on whom narcotic analgesics have been used during the birth, or who are drug addicts.
▲/ ✚ side-effects/warning: *see* NALOXONE.

***narcotic** is a somewhat confusing term that is properly applied to drugs that induce stupor and insensibility. Most commonly the term is used to describe OPIATES (such as MORPHINE and DIAMORPHINE), but logically it can also be used to describe SEDATIVES and HYPNOTIC drugs and alcohol, which act directly on the brain centres to depress their functioning. In law, however, the term describes an addictive drug that is the subject of abuse, including stimulant drugs, such as COCAINE (especially in the USA).

***narcotic analgesic:** *see* ANALGESIC.

Nardil (*Parke-Davis*) is a proprietary ANTIDEPRESSANT drug of the MAO INHIBITOR class, available only on prescription, used to treat depressive illness. Produced in the form of tablets, Nardil is a preparation of the potentially dangerous drug phenelzine (which requires a careful dietary regimen to accompany treatment because of complex interactions with various foods such as cheese, yeast extract, chocolate etc.). It is not recommended for children.
▲/ ✚ side-effects/warning: *see* PHENELZINE.

Narphen (*Smith & Nephew Pharmaceuticals*) is a proprietary, NARCOTIC ANALGESIC, a controlled OPIATE consisting of a preparation of phenazocine hydrobromide, used to relieve severe pain and pancreatic or biliary pain. Produced in the form of tablets, Narphen is not recommended for children.
▲/ ✚ side-effects/warning: *see* PHENAZOCINE.

nefopam is an non-narcotic ANALGESIC used to treat moderate to severe pain, such as that following surgery, or in cancer or toothache. Administration is oral in the form of tablets, or by injection.

▲ side-effects: there may be nausea, dry mouth, nervous agitation and insomnia. A few patients experience blurred vision, drowsiness, headache, an increase in the heart rate and sweating. Rarely, there is discoloration of the urine.

♣ warning: nefopam should not be administered to patients who suffer from convulsive disorders, or who are undergoing a heart attack. It should be administered with caution to those with certain types of glaucoma, liver disease or urinary retention. Not recommended for children.
Related article: ACUPAN.

Nepenthe (*Evans*) is a proprietary, NARCOTIC ANALGESIC, which, because it is a preparation of the OPIATES anhydrous morphine and opium tincture, is on the controlled drugs list. It is used to relieve severe pain, especially during the final stages of terminal malignant disease, it is produced in the form of a syrup for dilution (the potency of the syrup once dilute is retained for 4 weeks) and in ampoules for injection. Nepenthe solution is not recommended for children aged under 12 months; the injection is not recommended for children aged under 6 years.

▲/♣ side-effects/warning: *see* MORPHINE.

Neulactil (*May & Baker*) is an ANTIPSYCHOTIC drug, available only on prescription, used to treat and tranquillize patients who are undergoing behavioural disturbances, or who are psychotic (such as schizophrenia); it may also be used to treat severe anxiety in the short term. Produced in the form of tablets (in three strengths) and as a strong syrup for dilution (the potency of the syrup once dilute is retained for 14 days), Neulactil is a preparation of the antipsychotic drug pericyazine.

▲/♣ side-effects/warning: *see* PERICYAZINE.

Neurodyne (*Radiol*) is a proprietary, non-prescription, compound ANALGESIC, which is not available from the National Health Service. Used to treat pain anywhere in the body, Neurodyne is a preparation of paracetamol and the OPIATE codeine phosphate. Produced in the form of capsules, it is not recommended for children.

▲/♣ side-effects/warning: *see* CODEINE PHOSPHATE; PARACETAMOL.

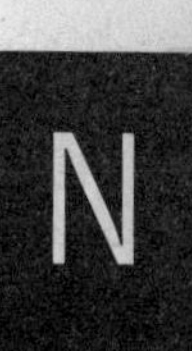

neuroleptic a term that was applied originally to the phenothiazine group of drugs in the early 1950s to describe their property of inducing a state of 'artificial hibernation', where a treated individual was not in a state of unconsciouness, but was clearly sedated and appeared to show little interest in what was going on. Major tranquillizer was another name given to drugs of this nature. These drugs were quickly recognized to be very effective antipsychotic agents and this term is more commonly used nowadays.
see ANTIPSYCHOTIC; TRANQUILLIZERS.

***neurotransmitters** are chemical messengers that, on excitation of the nerve, are released from nerve endings to act locally to excite or inhibit either other nerves or the cells within organs innervated by the nerves (such as the heart, intestine, skeletal muscle, or glands). Thus neurotransmitters are rather like HORMONES, but unlike the latter they act locally rather than on circulation in the blood. Examples include: ACETYLCHOLINE; DOPAMINE; NORADRENALINE; SEROTONIN.

Nicorette (*Lundbeck*) is a proprietary, sugar-free chewing gum containing nicotine. It is available on prescription (with counselling) to private patients trying to stop smoking.
- ✚ warning: it should not be used during pregnancy, and it should be given with caution to those with angina pectoris or coronary artery disease. If the gum is swallowed it may exacerbate a peptic ulcer or gastritis.

N

Night Nurse (*Beecham Health Care*) is a proprietary, non-prescription, cold relief preparation produced in the form of capsules. It contains the ANALGESIC paracetamol, ALCOHOL, the ANTITUSSIVE dextromethorphan and the ANTIHISTAMINE promethazine, which has a marked sedative activity.
- ▲/✚ side-effects/warning: *see* DEXTROMETHORPHAN; PARACETAMOL; PROMETHAZINE HYDROCHLORIDE.

nikethamide is a respiratory stimulant drug, used to relieve severe respiratory difficulties in patients who suffer from chronic disease of the respiratory tract, or who undergo respiratory depression following major surgery – particularly in cases where ventilatory support is not applicable. As a respiratory stimulant, however, nikethamide is now less commonly used. Administration is by slow intravenous injection, and may be repeated at intervals of between 15 and 30 minutes. It should only be given under expert supervision in a hospital.
- ▲ side-effects: there may be nausea, restlessness and tremor, leading possibly to convulsions and heartbeat irregularities.
- ✚ warning: nikethamide should not be administered to patients with respiratory failure resulting from drug overdose or neurological disease, or with coronary artery disease, severe asthma, or an excess of thyroid hormones in the blood (thyrotoxicosis). It should be administered with caution to those with severe high blood pressure (hypertension) or a reduced supply of blood to the heart. Effective dosage is unfortunately close to the level that causes toxic effects, especially convulsions.

Nitoman (*Roche*) is a proprietary preparation of the powerful drug tetrabenazine, available only on prescription, used to assist a patient to regain voluntary control of movement in Huntington's chorea and related disorders. It is thought to work by reducing the amount of the neurotransmitter DOPAMINE in the nerve endings of the brain. Produced in the form of tablets, Nitoman is not recommended for children.
- ▲/✚ side-effects/warning: *see* TETRABENAZINE.

nitrazepam is a comparatively mild HYPNOTIC drug, one of the BENZODIAZEPINES. It is used primarily in the short-term treatment of insomnia, in patients where a degree of sedation during the daytime is acceptable. However, nitrazepam is thought to be potentially habituating (addictive), and continuous use may in any case have cumulative effects, so many doctors now prefer to prescribe other shorter-acting benzodiazepines instead. Administration is oral in the form of tablets, as capsules, or as a suspension (mixture).

▲ side-effects: concentration and speed of reaction are affected. There is commonly drowsiness; there may also be sensitivity reactions and, in the elderly, a mild state of confusion. Prolonged use may lead to tolerance and a form of dependence (in which there may be insomnia that is worse than before).

● warning: nitrazepam should be administered with caution to patients with certain diseases of the lungs (particularly if respiratory depression is a symptom), or who are pregnant or lactating. The dose should be reduced in those patients who are elderly or debilitated, who have impaired liver or kidney function. The consumption of alcohol enhances the hypnotic effect of the drug. Withdrawal of treatment should be gradual (abrupt withdrawal after prolonged use may give rise to withdrawal symptoms).
Related articles: MOGADON; REMNOS; SOMNITE; SUREM; UNISOMNIA.

nitrous oxide is a general ANAESTHETIC used to induce and maintain anaesthesia. It is used in conjunction with other general anaesthetics when lower dosages of other drugs can then be used. A mixture of nitrous oxide and oxygen may be administered to produce analgesia without loss of consciousness.

▲/● side-effects/warning: prolonged exposure to nitrous oxide may have harmful effects on blood components.

Nobrium (*Roche*) is a proprietary minor TRANQUILLIZER, available on prescription only to private patients, used in the short-term treatment of anxiety. Produced in the form of capsules (in two strengths), Nobrium is a preparation of the long-acting ANXIOLYTIC BENZODIAZEPINE medazepam. It is not recommended for children.

▲/● side-effects/warning: *see* MEDAZEPAM.

Noctec (*Squibb*) is a proprietary HYPNOTIC drug, available only on prescription, used to treat insomnia and for sedation in the elderly. Produced in the form of capsules, Noctec is a preparation of the powerful SEDATIVE chloral hydrate, and is not recommended for children.

▲/● side-effects/warning: *see* CHLORAL HYDRATE.

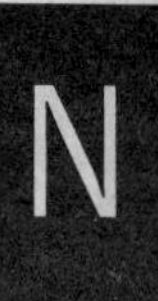

***non-narcotic analgesic:** *see* ANALGESIC.

***non-steroidal anti-inflammatory drug** is usually abbreviated to NSAID.
see ANALGESIC; ANTI-INFLAMMATORY.

noradrenaline is a NEUROTRANSMITTER and a HORMONE produced and secreted by peripheral sympathetic nerves, by many nerve fibres in the brain, and by the central core (medulla) of the adrenal glands. Like the closely related adrenaline, it represents a vital element in the sympathetic nervous system in that as a neurotransmitter it plays a major role in the body's response to stress. When stressed the body releases noradrenaline (and adrenaline) to organize constriction of the small blood vessels (vasoconstriction) so increasing blood pressure, which increases the rate and force of the heartbeat, and to relax the muscles of the intestinal wall. It is to effect one or more of these responses that noradrenaline, as a SYMPATHOMIMETIC, may be administered therapeutically. In an emergency, for example, noradrenaline (in the form of noradrenaline acid tartrate) may be injected to raise depressed blood pressure.

▲ side-effects: there may be headache, reduced heart rate and uneven heartbeat.

⯃ warning: noradrenaline should not be administered to patients who are undergoing a heart attack, or who are pregnant. Leakage of the hormone into the tissues at the site of injection may cause tissue damage.

N

nortriptyline is a TRICYCLIC ANTIDEPRESSANT drug, which also has mild sedative properties, used primarily to treat depressive illness. Like several others of its type, however, the drug may also be used to assist in the treatment of nocturnal bedwetting by children (aged over 7 years). Administration is oral in the form of tablets, capsules, or a sugar-free dilute liquid.

▲ side-effects: common effects include mild sedation (possibly affecting driving ability), dry mouth and blurred vision; there may also be difficulty in urinating, sweating and irregular heartbeat, behavioural disturbances, a rash, a state of confusion, and/or a loss of libido. Rarely, there are also blood disorders.

⯃ warning: nortriptyline should not be administered to patients who suffer from heart disease or psychosis; it should be administered with caution to patients who suffer from diabetes, epilepsy, liver or thyroid disease, glaucoma or urinary retention; or who are pregnant or lactating. Withdrawal of treatment must be gradual.

Related articles: ALLEGRON; AVENTYL.

Norval (*Bencard*) is a proprietary ANTIDEPRESSANT, available only on prescription, used to treat depressive illness especially when sedation is required. Produced in the form of tablets (in three strengths), Norval is a preparation of mianserin hydrochloride. It is not recommended for children.

▲/⯃ side-effects/warning: *see* MIANSERIN.

Nozinan (*Rhône-Poulenc Rorer*) is a proprietary ANTIPSYCHOTIC drug, available only on prescription, used to treat and sedate patients with schizophrenia and related psychoses, and to sedate and relieve anxiety during terminal care. Produced in ampoules for injection, Nozinan is a preparation of methotrimeprazine hydrochloride. It is not recommended for children.

▲/⯃ side-effects/warning: *see* METHOTRIMEPRAZINE.

***NSAID** is an abbreviation of non-steroidal ANTI-INFLAMMATORY drug.

see ANALGESIC; ANTIRHEUMATIC.

Nubain (*Du Pont*) is a proprietary, narcotic ANALGESIC, available only on prescription, used to treat moderate to severe pain, particularly during or following surgical procedures or a heart attack. Produced in ampoules for injection, Nubain is a preparation of the OPIATE nalbuphine hydrochloride. It is not recommended for children.

▲/⯃ side-effects/warning: *see* NALBUPHINE HYDROCHLORIDE.

Nurofen (*Crookes Healthcare*) is a proprietary, non-prescription, non-narcotic ANALGESIC containing ibuprofen.

▲/⯃ side-effects/warning: *see* IBUPROFEN.

Nu-Seals Aspirin (*Lilly*) is a proprietary, non-prescription, non-narcotic ANALGESIC, a form of aspirin used to treat chronic pain such as that of arthritis and rheumatism. Produced in the form of tablets (in two strengths), Nu-Seals Aspirin is not recommended for children aged under 12 years.

▲/ ● side-effects/warning: *see* ASPIRIN.

Nycopren (*Lundbeck*) is a proprietary, non-steroidal, ANTI-INFLAMMATORY (NSAID), non-narcotic ANALGESIC, available only on prescription, used to relieve pain – particularly rheumatic and arthritic pain, and that of acute gout – and to treat other musculo-skeletal disorders. Produced in the form of tablets (in two strengths), it is a preparation of naproxen.

▲/ ● side-effects/warning: *see* NAPROXEN.

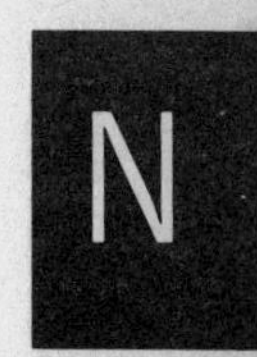

Omnopon (*Roche*) is a proprietary OPIATE, a controlled drug which is a preparation of papaveretum, used primarily as premedication before surgery, but also to relieve severe pain. It is produced in the form of ampoules for injection.
▲/✚ side-effects/warning: *see* PAPAVERETUM.

Omnopon-Scopolamine (*Roche*) is a proprietary combination of Omnopon and the powerful alkaloid SEDATIVE hyoscine (also known as scopolamine in the USA). It is a controlled drug, and is used primarily as pre-medication before surgery. It is produced in ampoules for injection.
▲/✚ side-effects/warning: *see* PAPAVERETUM; HYOSCINE.

O

ondansetron is a recently introduced ANTI-EMETIC drug, which gives relief from nausea and vomiting, especially in patients receiving radiotherapy and chemotherapy, and where other drugs are ineffective. It acts by preventing the action of the naturally-occuring HORMONE and NEUROTRANSMITTER SEROTONIN. It is used in those over 4 years of age, and is given as tablets or by slow intravenous injection or infusion
▲ side-effects: headache, constipation, warmth or flushing in the head and over stomach. Hypersensitivity reactions and effects on liver enzymes have been reported.
✚ warning: do not use in pregnancy or breast-feeding.
Related article: ZOFRAN.

opiates are a group of drugs, derived from opium, that depress certain functions of the central nervous system. In this way, they can relieve pain (and inhibit coughing). They are also used to treat diarrhoea. Therapeutically, the most important opiate is probably morphine which, with its synthetic derivative heroin (diamorphine), is a NARCOTIC; all are potentially habituating (addictive).
▲/✚ side-effects/warning: *see* BUPRENORPHINE; CODEINE PHOSPHATE; DEXTROMORAMIDE; DIAMORPHINE; DIHYDROCODEINE TARTRATE; MEPTAZINOL; METHADONE; MORPHINE; PAPAVERETUM; PENTAZOCINE; PETHIDINE; PHENAZOCINE.

opiate squill linctus and pastilles are compound formulations not available from the National Health Service, combining several soothing liquids – including camphorated tincture of opium and tolu syrup – into a cough linctus (also known as Gee's linctus) and into a form of cough pastilles (also known as Gee's pastilles) made from that linctus.

opium alkaloids is another term for opiates.
see OPIATES.

Oramorph (*Boehringer Ingelheim*) is a proprietary NARCOTIC ANALGESIC. It is used primarily to relieve pain following surgery, or the pain experienced during the final stages of terminal malignant disease. Produced in the form of an oral solution in two strengths, the more concentrated of which is on the controlled drugs list. It is a preparation of the OPIATE and narcotic morphine sulphate; it is not recommended for children.
▲/✚ side-effects/warning: *see* MORPHINE.

Orap (*Janssen*) is a proprietary ANTIPSYCHOTIC, available only on prescription, used with care to treat and tranquillize patients who are psychotic, particularly schizophrenic. It should not be

used unless there is evidence of a healthy ECG. Produced in the form of tablets (in three strengths), Orap is a preparation of pimozide.
▲/✚ side-effects/warning: *see* PIMOZIDE.

orphenadrine hydrochloride is an ANTICHOLINERGIC drug used primarily to treat the symptoms of parkinsonism (whether drug-induced or not) and drug induced extrapyramidal symptoms (*see* ANTIPARKINSONIAN). It thus reduces tremor and rigidity, has a diuretic effect on the excess salivary flow, but can do little to improve slowness or awkwardness in movement. Administration of orphenadrine hydrochloride is oral in the form of tablets or as an elixir, or by injection.
▲ side-effects: there may be dry mouth, urinary retention and gastrointestinal disturbances; visual disturbances may also arise, with dizziness. Rarely, there is increased heart rate and/or a hypersensitivity reaction, mental confusion and nervousness.
✚ warning: prolonged use can reduce muscle tone in an affected muscle, leading eventually to worse disability. The drug should be administered with caution to patients with heart, kidney or liver disease, glaucoma, gastrointestinal obstruction or urinary retention. Withdrawal of treatment must be gradual. It should not be administered to children.
Related articles: BIORPHEN; DISIPAL.

Orudis (*May & Baker*) is a proprietary, ANTI-INFLAMMATORY, non-narcotic ANALGESIC, available only on prescription, used to relieve arthritic and rheumatic pain and to treat other musculo-skeletal disorders. Produced in the form of capsules (in two strengths) and as anal suppositories, Orudis's active constituent is ketoprofen.
▲/✚ side-effects/warning: *see* KETOPROFEN.

Oruvail (*May & Baker*) is a proprietary, ANTI-INFLAMMATORY, non-narcotic ANALGESIC, available only on prescription, used to relieve arthritic and rheumatic pain and to treat other musculo-skeletal disorders. Produced in the form of capsules (in two strengths), and as ampoules for injection, Oruvail's active constituent is ketoprofen.
▲/✚ side-effects/warning: *see* KETOPROFEN.

Oxanid (*Steinhard*) is a proprietary ANXIOLYTIC or TRANQUILLIZER drug, available only on prescription to private patients. It is used for treating anxiety in the short-term only because dependence may occur. Produced in the form of tablets (in three strengths), Oxanid is a preparation of the BENZODIAZEPINE oxazepam.
▲/✚ side-effects/warning: *see* OXAZEPAM.

oxazepam is a short-acting ANXIOLYTIC or TRANQUILLIZER drug, one of the BENZODIAZEPINES used primarily to relieve anxiety. It causes less drowsiness the next day because it is short-acting, and is therefore useful in the elderly. However, oxazepam is not suitable for prolonged use because dependence may occur. Administration is oral in the form of tablets or capsules.
▲ side-effects: drowsiness usually occurs; there may also be unsteadiness, headache, and shallow breathing. Hypersensitivity reactions may occur. Repeated doses are, however, less cumulative in

O

effect than with many other benzodiazepine anxiolytics.

- warning: oxazepam may reduce a patient's concentration and intricacy of movement or thought; it may enhance the effects of alcohol consumption. Prolonged use or abrupt withdrawal should be avoided. It should be administered with caution to patients with respiratory difficulties, glaucoma, or kidney or liver damage; who are in the last stages of pregnancy; or who are elderly or debilitated.
Related article: OXANID.

O

oxypertine is an ANTIPSYCHOTIC drug used to treat psychosis (such as in schizophrenia); it is suitable both for manic and hyperactive forms of behavioural disturbance, as well as for apathetic and withdrawal forms. The drug may also be used to treat severe anxiety in the short term. Extrapyramidal motor disorders are less likely with this drug than with some other antipsychotics. Administration is oral in the form of capsules or tablets.

▲ side-effects: extrapyramidal motor disorders may occur with high dosage. Patients should be warned before treatment that their judgement and powers of concentration may become defective under treatment. Low doses may cause agitation and high doses sedation.

- warning: oxypertine should not be administered to patients who suffer from reduction in the bone marrow's capacity for producing blood cells, or from certain types of glaucoma. It should be administered only with caution to patients with heart or vascular disease, kidney or liver disease, parkinsonism, or depression; or who are pregnant or lactating. Abrupt withdrawal should be avoided. It is not recommended for children.
Related article: INTEGRIN.

Pacifene (*Sussex Pharmaceuticals*) is a proprietary, non-narcotic, ANALGESIC containing ibuprofen, which also has ANTI-INFLAMMATORY properties (NSAID). It is available without prescription as tablets (in three strengths).
▲/ ♣ side-effects/warning: *see* IBUPROFEN.

Palaprin Forte (*Nicholas*) is a proprietary, non-prescription, ANTI-INFLAMMATORY, non-narcotic ANALGESIC used to relieve pain – particularly rheumatic and arthritic pain – and to treat other musculo-skeletal disorders. Produced in the form of tablets, Palaprin Forte is a preparation of the non-narcotic analgesic aloxipirin.
▲/ ♣ side-effects/warning: *see* ALOXIPIRIN.

Paldesic (*RP Drugs*) is a proprietary, non-prescription form of the non-narcotic ANALGESIC paracetamol. It is produced in the form of a syrup.
▲/ ♣ side-effects/warning: *see* PARACETAMOL.

Palfium (*Boehringer Mannheim*) is a proprietary, narcotic ANALGESIC, which, because it is a preparation of the OPIATE dextromoramide, is on the controlled drugs list. Used to relieve severe pain, especially during the final stages of terminal malignant disease, it is produced in the form of tablets (in two strengths), ampoules (in two strengths) for injection, and anal suppositories (which are not recommended for children).
▲/ ♣ side-effects/warning: *see* DEXTROMORAMIDE.

Pamergan P100 (*Martindale*) is a proprietary narcotic ANALGESIC on the controlled drugs list, used both in the relief of pain and as a premedication prior to surgery, especially obstetrics. Produced in ampoules for injection, Pamergan P100 is a preparation of the narcotic analgesic pethidine hydrochloride and the SEDATIVE ANTIHISTAMINE promethazine hydrochloride.
▲/ ♣ side-effects/warning: *see* PETHIDINE; PROMETHAZINE HYDROCHLORIDE.

Pameton (*Sterling Winthrop*) is a proprietary, non-prescription, non-narcotic ANALGESIC, not available from the National Health Service, used to treat pain (especially for patients likely to overdose) and to reduce high body temperature. Produced in the form of tablets, Pameton is a compound preparation of paracetamol and the amino acid METHIONINE (a paracetamol overdose antidote). It is not recommended for children aged under 6 years.
▲/ ♣ side-effects/warning: *see* METHIONINE; PARACETAMOL.

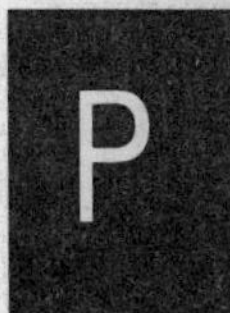

Panadeine (*Winthrop*) is a proprietary, non-prescription, compound ANALGESIC, not available from the National Health Service, used to treat pain and to reduce high body temperature. Produced in the form of tablets, it is a preparation of paracetamol and codeine (a combination known as co-codamol), and is not recommended for children aged under 7 years.
▲/ ♣ side-effects/warning: *see* CODEINE PHOSPHATE; PARACETAMOL.

Panadol (*Winthrop*) is a proprietary, non-prescription, non-narcotic ANALGESIC. Used to treat pain and to reduce high body temperature, it is produced in the form of tablets (of two kinds), as effervescent tablets (under the name Panadol Soluble), and as an elixir for dilution (the potency of the elixir once dilute is retained for 14 days). It is not available from the National Health Service. In all forms it is a preparation of paracetamol, and is not recommended for children aged under 3 months.

▲/✱ side-effects/warning: *see* PARACETAMOL.

Panaleve (*Leo*) is a proprietary form of the non-narcotic ANALGESIC paracetamol. Available without prescription, it is produced as an elixir.

▲/✱ side-effects/warning: *see* PARACETAMOL.

papaveretum is a compound preparation of alkaloids of opium, about half of which is made up of MORPHINE, the rest consisting of proportions of CODEINE, noscapine and PAPAVERINE. It is used as a NARCOTIC ANALGESIC primarily during or following surgery, but also as a SEDATIVE prior to an operation. Administration is oral in the form of tablets, or by injection. All proprietary preparations containing papaveretum are on the controlled drugs list: the drug is potentially addictive.

▲ side-effects: there is constipation and urinary retention, shallow breathing and cough suppression; there may also be nausea and vomiting, and drowsiness. Injections may cause pain and tissue damage at the site. Tolerance and dependence (addiction) occur readily.

✱ warning: papaveretum should not be administered to patients who are suffering from head injury or raised intracranial pressure; it should be administered with caution to those with asthma, impaired kidney or liver function, hypotension (low blood pressure), or hypothyroidism (underactivity of the thyroid gland), who are pregnant or breast-feeding, or who have a history of drug abuse. Dosage should be reduced for elderly or debilitated patients.
Related articles: OMNOPON; OMNOPON-SCOPOLAMINE.

papaverine is an alkaloid of opium, technically an OPIATE, but it is unlike many others in being primarily a SMOOTH MUSCLE RELAXANT, and having little or no ANALGESIC effect. It is consequently used mostly in the treatment of the bronchospasm of asthma or to relieve other spasmodic conditions of smooth muscle, such as in indigestion or in vascular disorders of the limbs. It is present in some cough preparations. Administration is mostly (in the form of papaverine hydrochloride) as a solution for an aerosol spray or as a linctus, in combination with other anti-asthma drugs; it may sometimes be prescribed in the form of tablets.

▲ side-effects: it may cause heartbeat irregularities, gastrointestinal disturbances, headache, sweating, vertigo and skin rash.

✱ warning: papaverine should not be administered to patients with heart disease, especially if it involves heartbeat irregularities, or glaucoma.
Related articles: PAVACOL-D; PHOLCOMED;

paracetamol is a non-narcotic ANALGESIC used to treat all forms of mild to moderate pain; although it is also effective in reducing high body temperature it has no capacity for relieving inflammation. In many ways it is similar to ASPIRIN – except that it does not cause gastric irritation. It may (in high overdosage or prolonged use) cause liver damage. Many proprietary

P

preparations combine the two analgesics (compound analgesics) although these are not generally recommended. Administration is oral in the form of tablets, capsules or a liquid.

▲ side-effects: there are few side-effects if dosage is low; high overdosage or prolonged use may result in liver dysfunction.

● warning: paracetamol should be administered with caution to patients with impaired liver function or who suffer from alcoholism (which causes liver damage).

Related articles: CAFADOL; CALPOL; CO-CODAMOL; CO-DYDRAMOL; CO-PROXAMOL; COSALGESIC; DISPROL; DISTALGESIC; FORMULIX; LOBAK; MEDISED; MEDOCODENE; MIDRID; MIGRALEVE; MYOLGIN; NEURODYNE; PAEDO-SED; PALDESIC; PAMETON; PANADEINE; PANADOL; PANALEVE; PARACLEAR; PARACODOL; PARADEINE; PARAHYPON; PARAKE; PARAMAX; PARAMOL; PARDALE; PAXALGESIC; PROPAIN; SALZONE; SOLPADEINE; SOLPADOL; SYNDOL; TYLEX; UNIFLU PLUS GREGOVITE C; UNIGESIC; VEGANIN.

Paraclear (*Sussex Pharmaceuticals*) is a proprietary, non-prescription, non-narcotic ANALGESIC produced in the form of soluble tablets. It contains paracetamol.

▲/● side-effects/warning: *see* PARACETAMOL.

Paracodol (*Fisons*) is a proprietary, non-prescription, compound ANALGESIC, not available from the National Health Service. Used to treat muscular and rheumatic pain, and produced in the form of tablets for effervescent solution, it is a preparation of paracetamol and codeine phosphate (a combination itself known as co-codamol) and is not recommended for children aged under 6 years.

▲/● side-effects/warning: *see* CODEINE; PARACETAMOL.

Paradeine (*Scotia*) is a proprietary, non-prescription compound ANALGESIC, not available from the National Health Service. Used to treat muscular and rheumatic pain, and produced in the form of tablets, Paradeine is a preparation of paracetamol and codeine phosphate, together with the laxative phenolphthalein.

▲/● side-effects/warning: *see* CODEINE PHOSPHATE; PARACETAMOL.

Parahypon (*Calmic*) is a proprietary, non-prescription compound ANALGESIC, not available from the National Health Service. Used to relieve most types of pain, and produced in the form of tablets, Parahypon is a preparation of paracetamol and codeine phosphate (CO-CODAMOL) with the STIMULANT caffeine. It is not recommended for children aged under 6 years.

▲/● side-effects/warning: *see* CAFFEINE; CODEINE PHOSPHATE; PARACETAMOL.

Parake (*Galen*) is a proprietary, non-prescription compound ANALGESIC, not available from the National Health Service. Used both to relieve pain and to reduce high body temperature, and produced in the form of tablets, Parake is a preparation of paracetamol and codeine phosphate (a combination itself known as co-codamol) and is not recommended for children.

▲/● side-effects/warning: *see* CODEINE PHOSPHATE; PARACETAMOL.

paraldehyde is a strong-smelling and fast-acting SEDATIVE. It is primarily used in the treatment of severe and continuous epileptic seizures (status epilepticus). It is generally administered by injection, although it is sometimes administered via the rectum in the form of an enema.

▲ side-effects: a rash is not uncommon. The injections may be painful.

⬢ warning: paraldehyde should be administered with caution to patients with lung disease or impaired liver function. Keep away from rubber, plastics or fabric.

P

Paramax (*Beecham*) is a proprietary, non-narcotic, ANALGESIC, available only on prescription, used to relieve the pain of migraine. Produced in the form of tablets and as a sugar-free powder in sachets for effervescent solution, Paramax is a preparation of the analgesic paracetamol and the ANTINAUSEANT metoclopramide hydrochloride. It is not recommended for children.

▲/⬢ side-effects/warning: *see* METOCLOPRAMIDE; PARACETAMOL.

Paramol (*Duncan, Flockhart*) is a proprietary compound ANALGESIC, available only on prescription to private patients, used as a painkiller and as a cough suppressant. Produced in the form of tablets, Paramol is a preparation of paracetamol and the OPIATE dihydrocodeine tartrate (a combination itself known as CO-DYDRAMOL) and is not recommended for children.

▲/⬢ side-effects/warning: *see* DIHYDROCODEINE TARTRATE; PARACETAMOL.

Pardale (*Martindale*) is a proprietary, non-prescription compound ANALGESIC, not available from the National Health Service. Used to relieve headaches and menstrual and rheumatic pain, and produced in the form of tablets, Pardale is a preparation of paracetamol and codeine phosphate (CO-CODAMOL) together with the mild STIMULANT caffeine hydrate. It is not recommended for children.

▲/⬢ side-effects/warning: *see* CAFFEINE; CODEINE PHOSPHATE; PARACETAMOL.

Parlodel (*Sandoz*) is a proprietary preparation of the drug bromocriptine, used primarily to treat parkinsonism but not the parkinsonian symptoms caused by certain drug therapies (*see* ANTIPARKINSONIAN). It is produced in the form of tablets (in two strengths) and capsules (in two strengths).

▲/⬢ side-effects/warning: *see* BROMOCRIPTINE.

Parmid (*Lagap*) is a proprietary ANTINAUSEANT, available only on prescription, used to treat severe conditions of nausea and vomiting especially when associated with gastrointestinal disorders, during radiotherapy, or accompanying treatment with cytotoxic drugs. Produced in the form of tablets, as a syrup, and in ampoules for injection, Parmid is a preparation of metoclopramide hydrochloride. Use is usually restricted to patients over 20 years of age.

▲/⬢ side-effects/warning: *see* METOCLOPRAMIDE.

Parnate (*Smith Kline & French*) is a proprietary ANTIDEPRESSANT drug, available only on prescription. Produced in the form of tablets, Parnate is a preparation of the MAO INHIBITOR tranylcypromine. It is not recommended for children.

▲/⬢ side-effects/warning: *see* TRANYLCYPROMINE.

Parstelin (*Smith Kline & French*) is a proprietary ANTIDEPRESSANT drug, available only on prescrip-

tion, used to treat depressive illness particularly in association with anxiety. Produced in the form of tablets, Parstelin is a compound preparation of the MAO INHIBITOR tranylcypromine and the tranquillizer trifluoperazine. It is not recommended for children.
▲/ ● side-effects/warning: *see* TRANYLCYPROMINE; TRIFLUOPERAZINE.

Pavacol-D (*Boehringer Ingelheim*) is a proprietary, non-prescription cough mixture. It is a sugar-free preparation of the OPIATES papaverine hydrochloride and pholcodine for solution with the sugar-substitute sorbitol (the potency of the mixture once dilute is retained for 14 days). It is not recommended for children aged under 12 months.
▲/ ● side-effects/warning: *see* PAPAVERINE; PHOLCODINE.

Paxalgesic (*Steinhard*) is a proprietary ANALGESIC available only on prescription to private patients. Used to relieve pain anywhere in the body, and produced in the form of tablets, Paralgesic is a preparation of the narcotic-like analgesic dextropropoxyphene together with paracetamol. This compound combination is known as co-proxamol). It is not recommended for children.
▲/ ● side-effects/warning: *see* CO-PROXAMOL; DEXTROPROPOXYPHENE; PARACETAMOL.

Paxane (*Steinhard*) is a proprietary HYPNOTIC, available on prescription only to private patients. It is used in the short-term treatment of insomnia in cases where some degree of daytime sedation is acceptable. Produced in the form of capsules (in two strengths), Paxane is a preparation of the long-acting BENZODIAZEPINE flurazepam. Prolonged use may result in dependence.
▲/ ● side-effects/warning: *see* FLURAZEPAM.

Paxofen (*Steinhard*) is a proprietary, ANTI-INFLAMMATORY, non-narcotic ANALGESIC, available only on prescription, used to treat the pain of rheumatic and other musculo-skeletal disorders. Produced in the form of tablets (in three strengths), Paxofen is a preparation of ibuprofen.
▲/ ● side-effects/warning: *see* IBUPROFEN.

pemoline is a fairly mild STIMULANT that works by direct action on the brain, and is used primarily in hyperactive children. Administration is oral in the form of tablets, it is not recommended and should not be used to treat depression.
▲ side-effects: concentration and speed of thought and movement may be affected. There may also be sweating, insomnia, restlessness, nervousness, night terrors, euphoria, depression, and headache. High dosage may cause heartbeat irregularities and dizziness, insomnia. agitation.
● warning: pemoline should not be administered to patients with heart disease, glaucoma, extrapyramidal disorders, hyperexcitable states or hypertension. Childrens' growth should be monitored. *Related article:* VOLITAL.

pentazocine is a powerful narcotic ANALGESIC used to treat moderate to severe pain. Much like MORPHINE in effect and action, it is less likely to cause dependence. Administration is oral in the form of capsules and tablets, topical in the form of anal suppositories, or by injection. Treatment by injection has a stronger effect than oral treatment. The proprietary form is on the controlled drugs list.

▲ side-effects: there is sedation and dizziness, with nausea; injection may lead to hallucinations. There is often also constipation. Tolerance and dependence (addiction) may result from prolonged treatment. There may also be hallucinations.

● warning: pentazocine should not be administered to patients who have recently had a heart attack, with high blood pressure (hypertension), porphyria, heart failure, respiratory depression or head injury, who are taking any other narcotic analgesic, who are pregnant or have kidney or liver damage. Patients should be warned that hallucinations and other disturbances in thought and sensation may occur, especially following administration by injection. *Related article:* FORTRAL.

pericyazine is an ANTIPSYCHOTIC drug, of the PHENOTHIAZINE class, used to tranquillize patients suffering from schizophrenia and other psychoses, particularly during behavioural disturbances. The drug may also be used in the short-term to treat severe anxiety. It is less likely to cause extrapyramidal motor disorders than many other antipsychotics, but is more sedative. Administration is oral in the form of tablets or a dilute elixir.

▲ side-effects: concentration and speed of thought and movement are affected; the effects of alcohol consumption are increased. There may be dry mouth and blocked nose, constipation and difficulty in urinating, and blurred vision; menstrual disturbances in women or impotence in men may occur, with weight gain; there may be sensitivity reactions. Some patients feel cold and depressed, and tend to suffer from poor sleep patterns. Blood pressure may be low and the heartbeat irregular. Prolonged high dosage may cause opacity in the cornea and lens of the eyes, and a purple pigmentation of the skin. Treatment by intramuscular injection may be painful.

● warning: pericyazine should not be administered to patients with certain forms of glaucoma, whose blood-cell formation by the bone-marrow is reduced, or who are taking drugs that depress certain centres of the brain and spinal cord. It should be administered with caution to those with lung disease, cardiovascular disease, epilepsy, parkinsonism, abnormal secretion by the adrenal glands, impaired liver or kidney function, undersecretion of thyroid hormones (hypothyroidism), enlargement of the prostate gland or any form of acute infection; who are pregnant or lactating; or who are elderly. Prolonged use requires regular checks on eye function and skin pigmentation. Withdrawal of treatment should be gradual. *Related article:* NEULACTIL.

perphenazine is an ANTIPSYCHOTIC drug, of the PHENOTHIAZINE class, used to tranquillize patients suffering from schizophrenia and other psychoses, particularly during behavioural disturbances. The drug may also be used in the short term to treat severe anxiety, to soothe patients who are dying, as a premedication prior to surgery, and to remedy intractable hiccups. Alternatively, it may be used to relieve nausea and vertigo caused by disorders in the middle or inner ear. Administration is oral in the form of tablets, or by injection.

▲ side-effects: extrapyramidal motor disorders (muscle spasms, tremor, restlessness) are relatively common and prolonged use may cause tardive dyskinesias. Concentration and speed of thought and movement are affected; the effects of alcohol consumption may be increased. There may be menstrual disturbances in women or impotence in men, and weight gain; there may be sensitivity reactions. Blood pressure may be low and the heartbeat irregular. Prolonged high dosage may cause opacity in the cornea and lens of the eyes, and a purple pigmentation of the skin. Treatment by intramuscular injection may be painful.

● warning: perphenazine should not be administered to patients with certain forms of glaucoma, whose blood-cell formation by the bone-marrow is reduced, or who are taking drugs that depress certain centres of the brain and spinal cord. It should be administered with caution to those with lung disease, cardiovascular disease, epilepsy, parkinsonism, abnormal secretion by the adrenal glands, impaired liver or kidney function, undersecretion of thyroid hormones (hypothyroidism), enlargement of the prostate gland or any form of acute infection; who are pregnant or lactating; or who are elderly. Prolonged use requires regular checks on eye function and skin pigmentation. Withdrawal of treatment should be gradual. It should not be administered to children.

Related article: FENTAZIN; TRIPTAFEN.

Pertofran (*Geigy*) is a proprietary TRICYCLIC ANTIDEPRESSANT, available only on prescription. Produced in the form of tablets, Pertofran is a preparation of desipramine hydrochloride. It is not recommended for children.

▲/● side-effects/warning: *see* DESIPRAMINE HYDROCHLORIDE.

pethidine is a NARCOTIC ANALGESIC used primarily for the relief of moderate to severe pain, especially in labour and childbirth. Its effect is rapid and short-lasting, so its sedative properties are made use of only as a premedication prior to surgery or to enhance the effects of other anaesthetics during or following surgery. Administration (as pethidine hydrochloride) is oral in the form of tablets, or by injection. Proprietary forms are on the controlled drugs list.

▲ side-effects: shallow breathing, urinary retention, constipation and nausea are all fairly common; tolerance and dependence (addiction) are possible. There may also be drowsiness and pain at the site of injection. An overdose can cause convulsions.

● warning: pethidine should not be administered to patients with head injury or raised intracranial pressure; it should be administered with caution to those with impaired kidney or liver function, asthma, depressed respiration, insufficient secretion of thyroid hormones (hypothyroidism) or low blood pressure (hypotension), or who are pregnant (except during labour) or breast feeding. Dosage should be reduced for

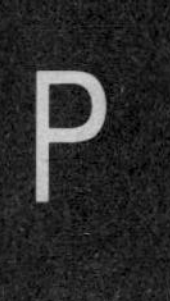

the elderly or debilitated.
Related articles: PAMERGAN P100; PETHILORFAN.

Pethilorfan (*Roche*) is a proprietary narcotic ANALGESIC on the controlled drugs list; it is used to treat moderate to severe pain, particularly in labour and childbirth. Produced in ampoules for injection, Pethilorfan is a preparation of pethidine hydrochloride with the respiratory stimulant levallorphan tartrate.
▲/● side-effects/warning: *see* PETHIDINE.

P

Phasal (*Lagab*) is a proprietary drug available only on prescription, used in the treatment and prevention of mania, and in the prevention of recurrent manic-depressive bouts. Produced in the form of sustained-release tablets, Phasal is a preparation of the drug lithium carbonate.
▲/● side-effects/warning: *see* LITHIUM.

phenazocine hydrobromide is a narcotic ANALGESIC used primarily for the relief of moderate to severe pain, especially pain arising from disorders of the pancreas or of the bile ducts. Administration (as phenazocine hydrobromide) is oral in the form of tablets. The proprietary form is on the controlled drugs list.
▲ side-effects: shallow breathing, urinary retention, constipation and nausea are all fairly common; tolerance and dependence (addiction) are possible. There may also be drowsiness.
● warning: phenazocine should not be administered to patients with head injury or raised intracranial pressure; it should be administered with caution to those with impaired kidney or liver function, asthma, depressed respiration, insufficient secretion of thyroid hormones (hypothyroidism) or low blood pressure (hypotension), or who are pregnant or lactating. Dosage should be reduced for the elderly or debilitated.
Related article: NARPHEN.

phenelzine is an ANTIDEPRESSANT drug, one of the MAO INHIBITORS. It is used particularly when treatment with TRICYCLIC antidepressants (such as AMITRIPTYLINE or IMIPRAMINE) has failed. Treatment with the drug requires a strict dietary regime – in which for example a patient must avoid eating cheese, or yeast extracts, or drinking alcohol – and extreme care in taking any other form of medication. Administration (as phenelzine sulphate) is oral in the form of tablets.
▲ side-effects: concentration and speed of thought and movement may be affected. There may also be dizziness, particularly on standing up from lying or sitting (because of low blood pressure). Much less commonly, there may be drowsiness (which may affect driving ability), rashes, sexual disturbances, headache, dry mouth and blurred vision, difficulty in urinating, constipation and a rash. Susceptible patients may experience agitation, tremor, or even psychotic episodes.
● warning: phenelzine should not be administered to patients with liver disease, epilepsy, porphyria, vascular disease of the heart or brain, or abnormal secretion of hormones by the adrenal glands, or who are children. It should be administered with caution to those who are elderly or debilitated, or who have diabetes mellitus, epilepsy, blood disorders or

cardiovascular disease. Counselling – if not supervision – over diet and any other medication is essential. Withdrawal of treatment should be gradual.
Related article: NARDIL.

Phenergan (*Rhône-Poulenc Rurer*) is a proprietary, non-prescription ANTIHISTAMINE. It is used because of its sedative properties to treat insomnia (especially in children) and in preoperative sedation in obstetrics and surgery. It also has ANTI-EMETIC properties. Phenergan is produced in the form of tablets (in two strengths), as an elixir for dilution (the potency of the elixir once dilute is retained for 14 days), neither of which is recommended for children aged under 6 months, and (only on prescription) in ampoules for injection, which is not recommended for children aged under 5 years. Phenergan is a preparation of promethazine hydrochloride. Under the name Phenergan Compound Expectorant, a compound linctus is also available, but not from the National Health Service, which consists of a preparation of promethazine hydrochloride and several LAXATIVE constituents; it too is not recommended for children aged under 5 years.
▲/✚ side-effects/warning: *see* PROMETHAZINE HYDROCHLORIDE.

phenobarbitone is a BARBITURATE, used in the prevention of recurrent epileptic seizures or the treatment of febrile convulsions. In all uses, prolonged treatment may rapidly result in tolerance and then dependence (addiction). Its use may also cause behavioural disturbances (such as hyperactivity) in children. Administration (as phenobarbitone or phenobarbitone sodium) is oral in the form of tablets and an elixir, or by injection. All proprietary preparations containing phenobarbitone are on the controlled drugs list. Although previously used as a HYPNOTIC and an ANXIOLYTIC it is rarely used now for these purposes.
▲ side-effects: there is drowsiness and lethargy; sometimes there is also depression, muscle weakness and/or sensitivity reactions in the form of skin rashes or blood disorders. Elderly or juvenile patients may experience psychological disturbance.
✚ warning: phenobarbitone should not be administered to patients with porphyria or who are already taking drugs that depress brain function (such as alcohol) on a regular basis; it should be administered with caution to those with impaired kidney or liver function, or who have respiratory disorders, who are elderly or children, or who are lactating. Withdrawal of treatment should be gradual.
Related article: GARDENAL SODIUM.

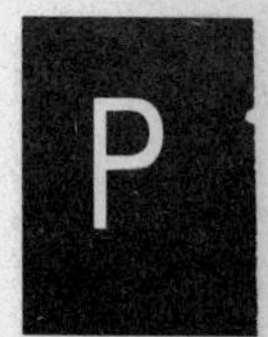

phenothiazine derivatives, or phenothiazines, are a group of drugs that are chemically related, but are not restricted to a single mode of activity. Many are ANTIPSYCHOTIC drugs, including some of the best-known and most-used, such as chlorpromazine, promazine, thioridazine, fluphenazine and trifluoperazine. Some of these are used also as ANTI-EMETICS. Others, such as piperazine, are ANTHELMINTICS.
▲/✚ side-effects/warning: *see* CHLORPROMAZINE; FLUPHENAZINE; METHOTRIMEPRAZINE; PERICYAZINE; PERPHENAZINE;

PIPOTHIAZINE; PROCHLORPERAZINE; PROMAZINE HYDROCHLORIDE; THIORIDAZINE; TRIFLUOPERAZINE.

Phensedyl (*May & Baker*) is a proprietary, non-prescription ANTITUSSIVE, which is not available from the National Health Service. Produced in the form of a linctus, Phensedyl is a preparation of the ANTIHISTAMINE promethazine hydrochloride, the OPIATE codeine phosphate and the SYMPATHOMIMETIC ephedrine hydrochloride as a syrup for dilution (the potency of the syrup once dilute is retained for 14 days). It is not recommended for children aged under 2 years.
▲/♣ side-effects/warning: *see* CODEINE PHOSPHATE; PROMETHAZINE HYDROCHLORIDE.

Phensic (*Beecham Health Care*) is a proprietary, non-prescription ANALGESIC containing aspirin and the STIMULANT caffeine.
▲/♣ side-effects/warning: *see* ASPIRIN; CAFFEINE.

phentermine is a SYMPATHOMIMETIC drug used under medical supervision and on a short-term basis to aid weight loss in moderate to severe obesity because it acts as an APPETITE SUPPRESSANT. Administration is in the form of sustained-release capsules.
▲ side-effects: there is commonly rapid heart rate, nervous agitation and insomnia, tremor, gastrointestinal disturbance, dry mouth, dizziness and headache.
♣ warning: phentermine should not be administered to patients who suffer from glaucoma; it should be administered with caution to those with heart disease, diabetes, epilepsy, peptic ulcer, or depression.
Related articles: DUROMINE; IONAMIN.

phenylbutazone is an ANTI-INFLAMMATORY, non-narcotic ANALGESIC, which, because of its sometimes severe side-effects, is used solely in the treatment of progressive fusion of the synovial joints of the spine (ankylosing spondylitis) under medical supervision in hospitals. Even for that purpose, it is used only when all other therapies have failed. Treatment then, however, may be prolonged. Administration is oral in the form of tablets.
▲ side-effects: there may be gastrointestinal disturbances, nausea, vomiting, and allergic reactions such as a rash. Less often, there is inflammation of the glands of the mouth, throat and neck; pancreatitis, nephritis or hepatitis; or headache and visual disturbances. Rarely, there is severe fluid retention (which may eventually in susceptible patients precipitate heart failure) or serious and potentially dangerous blood disorders.
♣ warning: phenylbutazone should not be administered to patients with cardiovascular disease, thyroid disease, or impaired liver or kidney function; who are pregnant; or who have a history of stomach or intestinal haemorrhaging. It should be administered with caution to those who are elderly or lactating. Regular and frequent blood counts are essential.
Related articles: BUTACOTE; BUTAZONE.

phenytoin is an ANTICONVULSANT drug that is also an anti-arrhythmic. It is consequently used to treat several forms of epilepsy, including grand mal

P

(tonic-clonic seizures) and temporal lobe epilepsy, but not absence seizures, and to regularize the heartbeat (especially following the administration of a heart stimulant). The drug is also useful in assisting in the treatment of the neuropathy that sometimes accompanies diabetes, and when given alone or with carbamazepine to treat trigeminal neuralgia. Administration (as phenytoin or phenytoin sodium) is oral in the form of tablets, chewable tablets, capsules and a suspension, or by injection.

▲ side-effects: the heart rate and blood pressure are reduced; asystole (a 'missed beat') may occur. The skin and facial features may coarsen during prolonged treatment; there may also be acne, enlargement of the gums, and/or growth of excess hair. Some patients enter a state of confusion. Nausea and vomiting, headache, blurred vision, blood disorders and insomnia may occur.

⬢ warning: phenytoin should not be administered to patients whose heart rate is excessively fast, who have heart block, liver damage or who have already been administered lignocaine hydrochloride. Monitoring of plasma concentration of the drug is essential in the initial treatment of epilepsy in order to establish an optimum administration level. Withdrawal should be gradual. Drug interactions are common. *Related articles:* EPANUTIN; EPANUTIN READY MIXED PARENTERAL.

pholcodine is an OPIATE that is used as an ANTITUSSIVE constituent in cough linctuses or syrups. Although its action on the cough centre of the brain resembles that of other opiates, it has no ANALGESIC effect.

▲ side-effects: there is commonly constipation. High or prolonged dosage may lead to respiratory depression.

⬢ warning: pholcodine should not be taken by patients with liver or kidney disease; it should be taken with caution by patients who suffer from asthma or have a history of drug abuse. *Related articles:* COPHOLCO; EXPULIN; GALENPHOL; PAVACOL-D; PHOLCOMED.

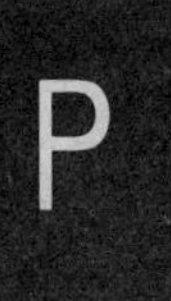

Pholcomed (*Medo*) is a proprietary brand of ANTITUSSIVES used to treat an irritable and unproductive cough. Produced in the form of a sugar-free linctus for use by diabetics (in two strengths, under the names Pholcomed-D and Pholcomed Forte Diabetic) and as pastilles (only the last of which preparations is available from the National Health Service), Pholcomed is a compound of the antitussive pholcodine and the smooth muscle relaxant papaverine hydrochloride, both of which are OPIATES. The Forte linctuses are not recommended for children.

▲/⬢ side-effects/warning: *see* PAPAVERINE; PHOLCODINE.

Pholcomed Expectorant (*Medo*) is a proprietary, non-prescription ANTITUSSIVE, which is not available from the National Health Service. It is a compound preparation of the expectorant guaiphenesin and the SYMPATHOMIMETIC methylephedrine hydrochloride.

Physeptone (*Calmic*) is a proprietary, narcotic ANALGESIC that is on the controlled drugs list. Used to treat severe pain, and produced in the form of tablets and in ampoules for injection,

Physeptone is a preparation of the OPIATE methadone hydrochloride; it is not recommended for children.
▲/ ● side-effects/warning: *see* METHADONE.

pimozide is an ANTIPSYCHOTIC drug, of the diphenylbutylpiperidine class, used to tranquillize patients suffering from schizophrenia and other psychoses including mania. It is especially effective in relieving hallucinations. The drug may also be used in the short-term to treat severe anxiety. It is less sedative than some antipsychotics, but it is more likely to cause extrapyramidal motor disorders. Administration is oral in the form of tablets.
▲ side-effects: extrapyramidal motor disorders (muscle spasms, tremor, restlessness) may occur and serious cardiac arrhythmias have been reported. Concentration and speed of thought and movement are affected; the effects of alcohol consumption are enhanced. There may be menstrual disturbances in women or impotence in men and with weight gain; there may be sensitivity reactions. Blood pressure may be low.
● warning: pimozide should not be administered to patients with a history, or evidence, of ECG abnormalities, whose blood-cell formation by the bone-marrow is reduced, or who are taking drugs that depress certain centres of the brain and spinal cord. It should be administered with caution to those with lung disease, cardiovascular disease, epilepsy, parkinsonism, abnormal secretion by the adrenal glands, impaired liver or kidney function, undersecretion of thyroid hormones (hypothyroidism), enlargement of the prostate gland or any form of acute infection; who are pregnant or lactating; or who are elderly. Prolonged use requires regular checks on eye function and skin pigmentation. Withdrawal of treatment should be gradual.
Related article: ORAP.

Piportil Depot (*May & Baker*) is a proprietary ANTIPSYCHOTIC drug, available only on prescription, used in maintenance therapy for patients who suffer from psychotic disorders such as chronic schizophrenia and related psychoses. Produced in ampoules for long-acting depot injections, Piportil Depot is a preparation of the PHENOTHIAZINE derivative pipothiazine palmitate; it is not recommended for children.
▲/ ● side-effects/warning: *see* PIPTHIAZINE PALMITATE.

pipothiazine palmitate is an ANTIPSYCHOTIC drug, one of the PHENOTHIAZINE derivatives used in maintenance therapy for patients who suffer from schizophrenia and other related psychoses. It appears likely to to have marked anticholinergic effects and a lower risk of extrapyramidal disorders than some other antipsychotics. Administration is by depot injection, designed for patients unable to take oral medication.
▲ side-effects: as a depot preparation side-effects are most likely to occur in the days immediately following injection. Extrapyramidal motor disorders, dry mouth, and difficulty in urination are likely to occur, as may constipation, eye problems and sedation.
● warning: it should be avoided in patients in a coma, who have arteriosclerosis, adrenal medullary tumours, renal failure, liver failure, cardiac

insufficiency, and hypersensitivity to other phenothiazines. It is not suitable for use in children, and it should be used with caution in those with narrow-angle glaucoma, respiratory disease, epilepsy, and thyroid disorders.
Related article: PIPORTIL DEPOT.

piroxicam is a non-steroidal, ANTI-INFLAMMATORY ANALGESIC (NSAID) used to treat pain and inflammation in rheumatic disease and other musculo-skeletal disorders (such as acute gout). Administration is oral in the form of capsules and soluble (dispersible) tablets, and topical in the form of anal suppositories.
▲ side-effects: there may be nausea and gastrointestinal disturbance, either or both of which may be reduced by taking the drug with milk or food. Some patients experience sensitivity reactions (such as headache, ringing in the ears – tinnitus – and vertigo), fluid retention, and/or blood disorders.
● warning: piroxicam should be administered with caution to patients with allergies, gastric ulceration or impaired liver or kidney function, or who are pregnant. Prolonged high dosage increases the risk of gastrointestinal disturbances.
Related articles: FELDENE; LARAPAM.

pizotifen is an ANTIHISTAMINE structurally related to tricyclic antidepressant drugs. It is used to treat and prevent headaches, particularly those in which blood pressure inside the blood vessels plays a part – such as migraine (*see* ANTIMIGRAINE). Administration is oral in the form of tablets and an elixir.
▲ side-effects: there may be drowsiness, dry mouth and blurred vision, with constipation and difficulty in urinating; sometimes there is muscle pain, dizziness, and/or nausea. Patients may put on weight.
● warning: pizotifen should be administered with care to patients with closed-angle glaucoma or urinary retention, or who are pregnant or lactating. The effects of alcohol may be enhanced.
Related article: SANOMIGRAN.

Ponderax (*Servier*) is a proprietary APPETITE SUPPRESSANT, available only on prescription, used as a short-term additional treatment in medical therapy for obesity. Produced in the form of sustained-release capsules ('Pacaps'), Ponderax is a preparation of the potentially addictive drug fenfluramine hydrochloride. It is not recommended for children.
▲/● side-effects/warning: *see* FENFLURAMINE HYDROCHLORIDE.

Ponstan (*Parke-Davis*) is a proprietary, ANTI-INFLAMMATORY, non-narcotic ANALGESIC (NSAID), available only on prescription, used to treat pain in rheumatoid arthritis, osteoarthritis and other musculo-skeletal disorders and period pain. Produced in the form of capsules, as tablets, as soluble (dispersible) tablets (under the name Ponstan Dispersible), and as a children's suspension for dilution (the potency of the suspension once dilute is retained for 14 days), Ponstan is a preparation of mefenamic acid. None of these products is recommended for children aged under 6 months.
▲/● side-effects/warning: *see* MEFENAMIC ACID.

Prepulsid (*Janssen*) is a stomach and intestine MOTILITY STIMULANT. It is a proprietary form of cisapride available only on

prescription, and available in the form of tablets which are taken 15–30 minutes before meals.
▲/✚ side-effects/warning: *see* CISAPRIDE.

Priadel (*Delandale*) is a proprietary drug, available only on prescription, used to treat acute mania and to prevent manic-depressive illness. Produced in the form of a sugar-free liquid, it is a preparation of lithium citrate. As lithium carbonate it is also available in tablet form. It is not recommended for children.
▲/✚ side-effects/warning: *see* LITHIUM.

prilocaine is primarily a local ANAESTHETIC, the drug of choice for very many topical or minor surgical procedures, especially in dentistry (because it is absorbed directly through mucous membranes). Administration is (in the form of a solution of prilocaine hydrochloride) by injection or topically as a cream.
▲ side-effects: there is generally a slowing of the heart rate and a fall in blood pressure. Some patients under anaesthetic become agitated, others enter a state of euphoria. Sometimes there is respiratory depression and convulsions.
✚ warning: prilocaine should not be administered to patients with the neural disease myasthenia gravis; it should be administered with caution to those with heart or liver failure (in order not to cause depression of the central nervous system and convulsions), or from epilepsy. Dosage should be reduced for the elderly and the debilitated. Full facilities for emergency cardio-respiratory resuscitation should be on hand during anaesthetic treatment.
Related articles: CITANEST; CITANEST WITH OCTAPRESSIN.

primidone is an ANTICONVULSANT drug used in the treatment of many forms of epilepsy (but not absence seizures) and of tremors due to old age or infirmity. It is converted in the body to the BARBITURATE phenobarbitone, and its actions and effects are thus identical to those of that drug.
▲/✚ side-effects/warning: *see* PHENOBARBITONE.
Related article: MYSOLINE.

Primperan (*Berk*) is a proprietary ANTINAUSEANT, available only on prescription, used to treat nausea and vomiting especially in gastrointestinal disorders, during treatment for cancer with cytotoxic drugs or radiotherapy, or in association with migraine. Produced in the form of tablets, as a sugar-free syrup for dilution (the potency of the syrup once dilute is retained for 14 days) and in ampoules for injection, Primperan is a preparation of metoclopramide hydrochloride. It is not recommended for children aged under 5 years.
▲/✚ side-effects/warning: *see* METOCLOPRAMIDE.

prochlorperazine is a PHENOTHIAZINE derivative used as an ANTIPSYCHOTIC drug in the treatment of psychosis (such as schizophrenia); as an ANXIOLYTIC in the short-term treatment of anxiety; and as an ANTI-EMETIC in the prevention of nausea caused by gastrointestinal disorder, by chemotherapy and radiotherapy in the treatment of cancer, or by the vertigo that results from disorders of the middle or inner ear. It is less sedative, but more likely to cause extrapyramidal motor disorders than some antipsychotics. Administration (as prochlorpromazine maleate or prochlorpromazine mesylate) is oral in the form of tablets, sustained-release capsules and syrups, in the form of anal suppositories, or by injection.

▲ side-effects: extrapyramidal motor disorders (muscle spasms, restlessness and tremor) may occur and with prolonged use there is a risk of tardive dyskinesias. Concentration and speed of thought and movement may be affected.

● warning: prochlorpromazine should not be administered to patients whose blood-cell formation by the bone-marrow is reduced, or who are taking drugs that depress certain centres of the brain and spinal cord. It should be administered with caution to those with lung disease, cardiovascular disease, epilepsy, parkinsonism, abnormal secretion by the adrenal glands, impaired liver or kidney function, undersecretion of thyroid hormones (hypothyroidism), enlargement of the prostate gland, or any form of acute infection; who are pregnant or lactating; or who are elderly. Prolonged treatment requires checks on eye function and skin pigmentation. Withdrawal of treatment should be gradual. *Related articles:* BUCCASTEM; STEMETIL; VERTIGON.

procyclidine is a powerful ANTICHOLINERGIC drug used to relieve some of the symptoms of parkinsonism, specifically the tremor of the hands, the overall rigidity of the posture, and the tendency to produce an excess of saliva. (The drug also has the capacity to treat these conditions in some cases where they are produced by drugs.) It is thought to work by compensating for the lack of dopamine in the brain that is the major cause of such parkinsonian symptoms. Administration – which may be in parallel with the administration of LEVODOPA – is oral in the form of tablets or a syrup or by injection.

▲ side-effects: there may be dry mouth, dizziness and blurred vision, and/or gastrointestinal disturbances. Some patients experience sensitivity reactions and anxiety. Rarely, and in susceptible patients, there may be confusion, agitation and psychological disturbance (at which point treatment may be withdrawn).

● warning: procyclidine should not be administered to patients who suffer not merely from tremor but from distinct involuntary movements; it should be administered with caution to those with impaired kidney or liver function, gastrointestinal obstruction, cardiovascular disease, closed-angle glaucoma, or urinary retention. Withdrawal of treatment must be gradual. *Related articles:* ARPICOLIN; KEMADRIN.

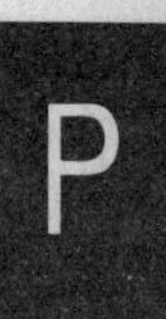

Proflex (*Lederle*) is a non-narcotic ANALGESIC drug with good ANTI-INFLAMMATORY (NSAID) properties. It is a proprietary form of ibuprofen. Available without prescription, it is used topically as a cream applied to the skin to treat the inflammatory symptoms of arthritis and to relieve soft tissue pain.

▲/● side-effects/warning: *see* IBUPROFEN.

Progesic (*Lilly*) is a proprietary, non-steroidal, ANTI-INFLAMMATORY, non-narcotic ANALGESIC (NSAID) used to relieve pain – particularly arthritic and rheumatic pain – and to treat other musculo-skeletal disorders. Available only on prescription, and produced in

the form of tablets, Progesic is a preparation of fenoprofen (as a calcium salt). It is not recommended for children.
▲/✚ side-effects/warning: *see* FENOPROFEN.

prolintane is a weak STIMULANT used as a constituent in some proprietary vitamin preparations, and intended to assist in the treatment of fatigue or lethargy. Prolonged or high dosage, however, may lead to a state of arousal and/or anxiety.
Related article: VILLESCON.

promazine hydrochloride is an ANTIPSYCHOTIC drug, of the PHENOTHIAZINE class, used to tranquillize agitated patients, especially patients who are elderly. The drug is also used in the short-term to treat severe anxiety, or to soothe patients who are dying. Administration is oral in the form of a suspension, or by injection.
▲ side-effects: extrapyramidal motor disorders are unlikely at the doses normally used. Concentration and speed of thought and movement are affected; the effects of alcohol consumption are enhanced. There may be dry mouth and blocked nose, constipation and difficulty in urinating, rash, jaundice and blurred vision; menstrual disturbances in women or impotence in men may occur, with weight gain; there may be sensitivity reactions. Blood pressure may be low and the heartbeat irregular. Treatment by intramuscular injection may be painful.
✚ warning: promazine hydrochloride should not be administered to patients with certain forms of glaucoma (closed-angle), whose blood-cell formation by the bone-marrow is reduced, or who are taking drugs that depress certain centres of the brain and spinal cord. It should be administered with caution to those with lung disease, cardiovascular disease, epilepsy, parkinsonism, abnormal secretion by the adrenal glands, impaired liver or kidney function, undersecretion of thyroid hormones (hypothyroidism), enlargement of the prostate gland or any form of acute infection; who are pregnant or lactating; or children. Prolonged use requires regular checks on eye function and skin pigmentation. Withdrawal of treatment should be gradual.
Related article: SPARINE.

promethazine hydrochloride is a powerful ANTIHISTAMINE that also has HYPNOTIC and ANTITUSSIVE properties. It is used also to induce sleep in the treatment of insomnia (especially in children) or as a premedication prior to surgery, and as a cough suppressant in cough linctuses. It may also be used in the treatment of parkinsonism, and as an ANTI-EMETIC in the prevention of nausea due to motion sickness or to ear infection. Its effect is comparatively long-lasting. Administration is oral in the form of tablets and a dilute elixir, or by injection.
▲ side-effects: concentration and speed of thought and movement may be affected. There may be headache, drowsiness and dry mouth, with gastrointestinal disturbances. Some patients experience blurred vision and/or sensitivity reactions on the skin.
✚ warning: promethazine should be administered with caution to patients with epilepsy, glaucoma, liver disease or enlargement of the prostate gland. During treatment, alcohol consumption must be avoided.

Related articles: Medised; Night Nurse; Pamergan P100; Phenergan; Phensedyl; Sominex.

promethazine theoclate is a salt of the powerful ANTIHISTAMINE promethazine, used primarily to prevent nausea and vomiting caused by motion sickness or infection of the ear. It is slightly longer-acting than the hydrochloride, but otherwise is similar in every respect.
▲/● side-effects/warning: *see* PROMETHAZINE HYDROCHLORIDE.
Related article: Avomine.

Prominal (*Winthrop*) is a proprietary form of the BARBITURATE methylpheno-barbitone, and is on the controlled drugs list. Produced in the form of tablets (in three strengths), Prominal is used to treat tonic-clonic and partial seizure epilepsy. It is not recommended for children.
▲/● side-effects/warning: *see* METHYLPHENOBARBITONE.

Prondol (*Wyeth*) is a proprietary ANTIDEPRESSANT drug, available only on prescription, used to treat depressive illness and associated symptoms. Produced in the form of tablets (in two strengths), Prondol is a preparation of the TRICYCLIC drug iprindole hydrochloride; it is not recommended for children.
▲/● side-effects/warning: *see* IPRINDOLE.

Propain (*Panpharma*) is a proprietary, non-prescription compound ANALGESIC, which is not available from the National Health Service. It is used to treat many forms of pain, including headache, migraine, muscular pain and menstrual problems. Produced in the form of tablets, Propain is a compound that includes the OPIATE codeine phosphate, the ANTIHISTAMINE diphenhydramine hydrochloride, the ANALGESIC paracetamol and the STIMULANT caffeine. It is not recommended for children.
▲/● side-effects/warning: *see* CAFFEINE; CODEINE PHOSPHATE; DIPHENHYDRAMINE HYDROCHLORIDE; PARACETAMOL.

Pro-Plus (*Ashe Consumer Products*) is a proprietary, non-prescription preparation of the STIMULANT caffeine for use in reducing fatigue.
▲/● side-effects/warning: *see* CAFFEINE.

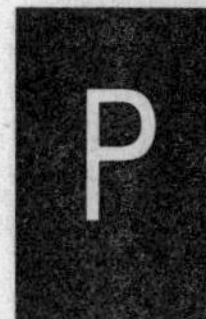

propofol is a general ANAESTHETIC used specifically for the initial induction of anaesthesia. Recovery after treatment is usually rapid and without any hangover effect. Administration is by injection.
▲ side-effects: there may sometimes be pain on injection, which can be overcome by prior administration of suitable premedication (such as a narcotic analgesic). Urine may turn green.
● warning: intravenous injection must be carried out with caution in order to avoid thrombophlebitis.
Related article: Diprivan.

propranolol is a BETA-BLOCKER used to treat migraine (*see* ANTIMIGRAINE, and it is also often used as an ANXIOLYTIC to relieve anxiety (particularly if there is tremor or palpitations). Administration (as propranolol hydrochloride) is oral in the form of tablets and sustained-release capsules, or by injection.
▲ side-effects: the heart rate is slowed; there may also be bronchospasm (causing asthma-like symptoms), gastrointestinal disturbances,

and tingling or numbness in the fingers and toes.

● warning: propranolol should not be administered to patients with any serious form of heart disease, or asthma. It should be administered with caution to those with impaired liver or kidney function, who are nearing the end of pregnancy, or who are lactating.
Related articles: BERKOLOL; INDERAL; SLOPROLOL.

Prothiaden (*Boots*) is a proprietary TRICYCLIC ANTIDEPRESSANT drug, available only on prescription, used to treat depressive illness especially in cases where some degree of sedation is deemed necessary. Produced in the form of tablets and capsules, Prothiaden is a preparation of dothiepin hydrochloride. It is not recommended for children.
▲/● side-effects/warning: *see* DOTHIEPIN HYDROCHLORIDE.

protriptyline is a TRICYCLIC ANTIDEPRESSANT drug used, because it has a stimulant effect, particularly to treat depressive illness that disposes towards apathy and withdrawal. Administration (as protriptyline hydrochloride) is oral in the form of tablets.

▲ side-effects: common effects include mild sedation (less than other antidepressants, but possibly affecting driving ability), dry mouth and blurred vision; anxiety, increased heart rate, agitation, rashes and hypotension are likely. There may also be difficulty in urinating, sweating, behavioural disturbances, a state of confusion, and/or a loss of libido. Rarely, there are also blood disorders.

● warning: protriptyline should not be administered to patients who suffer from heart disease or psychosis; it should be administered with caution to patients who suffer from diabetes, epilepsy, liver or thyroid disease, glaucoma or urinary retention; or who are pregnant or lactating. Withdrawal of treatment must be gradual.
Related article: CONCORDIN.

Prozac (*Dista*) is a proprietary form of the ANTIDEPRESSANT drug fluoxetine hydrochloride, which has less sedative effects than some drugs of this type. Available only on prescription, it is available as tablets.
▲/● side-effects/warning: *see* FLUOXETINE HYDROCHLORIDE.

quinalbarbitone sodium is a fast-acting BARBITURATE, used as a HYPNOTIC to promote sleep in conditions of severe intractable insomnia. It is a dangerous and potentially addictive drug, administered orally in the form of capsules. It is also used in the compound barbiturate Tuinal. All proprietary preparations containing quinalbarbitone sodium are on the controlled drugs list.

▲ side-effects: drowsiness, dizziness, lack of power to co-ordinate body movements (which may affect driving ability), shallow breathing and headache are all fairly common, especially in elderly patients. There may be allergic/sensitivity reactions.

● warning: quinalbarbitone sodium should not be administered to patients who have insomnia caused by pain, or porphyria, who are pregnant or lactating, or to the elderly or debilitated, or to children. In fact, usage should be avoided altogether where possible. It should be administered with caution to patients with respiratory difficulties, or liver or kidney disease. Tolerance, followed by dependence, occurs readily. Repeated doses have cumulative effect; abrupt withdrawal of treatment may precipitate serious withdrawal symptoms (including fits and delirium). It should not be used in patients with a history of alcohol abuse.

Related article: SECONAL SODIUM; TUINAL.

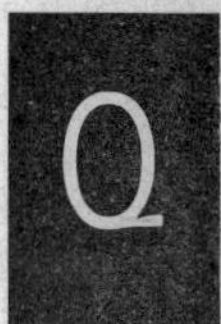

Rapifen (*Janssen*) is a proprietary ANALGESIC, which, because it is also a NARCOTIC, is on the controlled drugs list. It is used especially in outpatient surgery, short operational procedures, and for the enhancement of anaesthesia. Produced in the form of ampoules for injection, Rapifen is a preparation of alfentanil. A weaker paediatric injection is also available.
▲/ ✚ side-effects/warning: *see* ALFENTANIL.

Redeptin (*Smith Kline & French*) is a proprietary preparation of the ANTIPSYCHOTIC drug fluspirilene. Available only on prescription, it is used to treat psychoses. Produced in ampoules for long-acting injections, Redeptin is not recommended for children.
▲/ ✚ side-effects/warning: *see* FLUSPIRILENE.

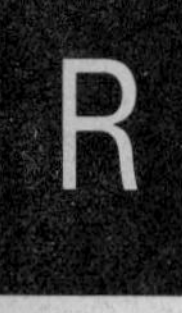

Relcofen (*Cox Pharmaceuticals*) is a proprietary, non-narcotic, ANALGESIC containing ibuprofen, which also has ANTI-INFLAMMATORY properties (NSAID). It is available without prescription as tablets (in three strengths).
▲/ ✚ side-effects/warning: *see* IBUPROFEN.

Relifex (*Bencard*) is a proprietary form of the non-steroidal, ANTI-INFLAMMATORY (NSAID) drug nabumetone. It is available on prescription as tablets and as a suspension to treat pain and inflammation in rheumatoid arthritis and osteoarthritis.
▲/ ✚ side-effects/warning: *see* NABUMETONE.

Remnos (*DDSA Pharmaceuticals*) is a proprietary TRANQUILLIZER and HYPNOTIC available on prescription only to private patients, used to treat insomnia in cases where some degree of daytime sedation is acceptable. Produced in the form of tablets (in two strengths), Remnos is a preparation of the long-acting BENZODIAZEPINE nitrazepam. It is potentially addictive.
▲/ ✚ side-effects/warning: *see* NITRAZEPAM.

Resolve (*Beecham Health Care*) is a proprietary, non-prescription formulation for the relief of 'morning after' hangover symptoms. Produced in the form of a powder, it contains citric acid, vitamin C, glucose, paracetamol and the ANTACIDS sodium carbonate, sodium bicarbonate and potassium bicarbonate.
▲/ ✚ side-effects/warning: *see* PARACETAMOL.

Revanil (*Roche*) is a recently introduced ANTIPARKINSONIAN drug, and is a proprietary form of lysuride maleate. Available only on prescription, the preparation is in the form of tablets.
▲/ ✚ side-effects/warning: *see* LYSURIDE MALEATE.

Rhumalgan (*APS, Cox, Kerfoot, Lagap*) is a proprietary form of the non-steroidal, ANTI-INFLAMMATORY (NSAID) drug diclofenac sodium. Available on prescription only as tablets (in two strengths) to treat pain and inflammation of musculo-skeletal disorders, such as rheumatic disease.
▲/ ✚ side-effects/warning: *see* DICLOFENAC SODIUM.

Rivotril (*Roche*) is a proprietary ANTICONVULSANT, available only on prescription, used to treat all forms of epilepsy. It is produced in the form of tablets (in two strengths) and in ampoules (with diluent) for injection, and is a preparation of the potentially addictive BENZODIAZEPINE clonazepam.

▲/ ● side-effects/warning: *see* CLONAZEPAM.

Robaxisal Forte (*Robins*) is a proprietary compound ANALGESIC, available on prescription only to private patients, used to relieve muscle spasm and pain, mainly in the muscles of the limbs; it works by direct action on the central nervous system. Produced in the form of tablets, Robaxisal Forte is a preparation of methocarbamol and aspirin. It is not recommended for children. Lower doses are recommended for the elderly.
▲/ ● side-effects/warning: *see* ASPIRIN.

Rohypnol (*Roche*) is a proprietary TRANQUILLIZER, available on prescription only to private patients, used for the short-term treatment of insomnia and sleep disturbance in cases where some degree of daytime sedation is acceptable. Produced in the form of tablets, Rohypnol is a preparation of the BENZODIAZEPINE flunitrazepam. It is not recommended for children. Prolonged use may result in dependence (addiction).
▲/ ● side-effects/warning: *see* FLUNITRAZEPAM.

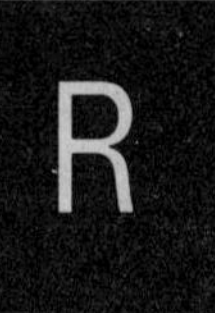

Sabril (*Merrell*) is an ANTI-EPILEPTIC drug, and is a proprietary form of vigabatrin available only on prescription, in the form of tablets.
▲/ ● side-effects/warning: *see* VIGABATRIN.

salsalate is a long-acting, non-narcotic ANALGESIC much like ASPIRIN, but without so many gastric side-effects, used primarily because of its ANTI-INFLAMMATORY properties to treat inflammation and pain in rheumatic and other musculo-skeletal disorders. Administration is oral in the form of capsules.
▲ side-effects: side-effects are not as common as they are with aspirin, but may include gastrointestinal disturbance or bleeding, hearing difficulties and ringing in the ears (tinnitus), and/or vertigo. There may also be sensitivity reactions, resulting in asthma-like symptoms and a rash.
● warning: salsalate should not be administered to patients who suffer from peptic ulcers, or who are aged under 12 years. It should be administered with caution to those with severely impaired function of the kidneys or the liver, or who are dehydrated; who are elderly; who have known allergies; who are pregnant or breast feeding; or who are already taking oral anticoagulant drugs.
Related article: DISALCID.

Salzone (*Wallace*) is a proprietary, non-prescription preparation of the non-narcotic ANALGESIC paracetamol, used to treat pain anywhere in the body. It is produced in the form of an elixir for dilution (the potency of the elixir once dilute is retained for 14 days).
▲/ ● side-effects/warning: *see* PARACETAMOL.

Sanomigran (*Sandoz*) is a proprietary preparation of the ANTIHISTAMINE pizotifen, a drug chemically related to some of the tricyclic antidepressants. It is used as an ANTIMIGRAINE drug because of its action on blood vessels in the head. Available only on prescription, and produced in the form of tablets (in two strengths) and as a sugar-free elixir, Sanomigran is not recommended for children aged under 5 years.
▲/ ● side-effects/warning: *see* PIZOTIFEN.

Scopoderm TTS (*Ciba*) is an ANTICHOLINERGIC and ANTI-NAUSEA drug, a proprietary form of hysocine hydrobromide, available only on prescription. It may be used to prevent motion sickness because of its ANTI-EMETIC properties. The preparation is available in the form of a special self-adhesive dressing that releases the active drug for absorption through the skin, usually a hairless site behind the ear. A single dressing should be put in place 5–6 hours before a journey, and can be replaced after 72 hours if necessary. The hands should be washed after application of the dressing.
▲/ ● side-effects/warning: *see* HYOSCINE.

scopolamine is another name for the powerful alkaloid drug hyoscine.
see HYOSCINE.

Sea-Legs (*Bioceuticals*) is a proprietary, non-prescription, anti-motion sickness preparation. It contains the ANTIHISTAMINE meclozine.
▲/ ● side-effects/warning: *see* MECLOZINE.

S

Seclodin (*Whitehall Laboratories*) is a proprietary, non-prescription, non-steroidal, ANTI-INFLAMMATORY, non-narcotic ANALGESIC preparation that contains ibuprofen.
▲/✚ side-effects/warning: *see* IBUPROFEN.

Seconal Sodium (*Lilly*) is a proprietary HYPNOTIC, a BARBITURATE on the controlled drugs list, which is used to treat intractable insomnia. Produced in the form of tablets (in two strengths), it is a preparation of amylobarbitone sodium.
▲/✚ side-effects/warning: *see* AMYLOBARBITONE SODIUM.

***sedatives** are drugs that calm and soothe, relieving anxiety and nervous tension, and disposing towards drowsiness. They are used particularly for premedication prior to surgery. Many are hypnotic drugs (such as BARBITURATES) used in doses lower than those administered to induce sleep.

selegiline is a drug that has the effect of inhibiting the enzyme that breaks down the neurotransmitter dopamine in the brain, and is accordingly used in combination with LEVODOPA (which is converted to dopamine in the brain) to treat the symptoms of parkinsonism (*see* ANTIPARKINSONIAN). In this way it supplements and extends the action of levodopa, also (in many patients) succesfully reducing some side-effects.
▲ side-effects: there may be nausea and vomiting, with agitation and hypotension (low blood pressure); some patients experience a state of confusion.
✚ warning: in some patients the side-effects are in fact aggravated by the combination of drugs, and the dosage of levodopa may have to be reduced.

Serc (*Duphar*) is a proprietary ANTI-EMETIC, available only on prescription, used to relieve symptoms of nausea caused by the vertigo and loss of balance experienced in infections of the middle and inner ears (such as Ménières disease). Produced in the form of tablets, Serc is a preparation of betahistine hydrochloride. It is not recommended for children.
▲/✚ side-effects/warning: *see* BETAHISTINE HYDROCHLORIDE.

Serenace (*Searle*) is a proprietary series of preparations of the ANTIPSYCHOTIC drug haloperidol, all available only on prescription, and used to treat most forms of mental disturbance from severe, short-term anxiety to long-term psychosis (including schizophrenia and mania, in emergency and maintenance modes of treatment). Serenace is produced as tablets (in four strengths), as capsules, as a liquid for swallowing, and in ampoules for injection (in two strengths). In all forms except that of the liquid, Serenace is not recommended for children.
▲/✚ side-effects/warning: *see* HALOPERIDOL.

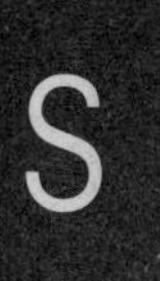

serotonin is an amine (5-hydroxytryptamine or 5-HT) that has a number of different roles in the body. In the brain important nerve tracts releasing serotonin as their NEUROTRANSMITTER are thought to be involved in aspects of brain function, such as different sleep states, temperature regulation, perception of pain, and mood control. Until recently little was known of the way in which serotonin acted in the brain, but the arrival of novel drugs acting on specific serotonin receptors hold much promise for the understanding of its mechanisms of action. Drugs

affecting serotoninergic systems include: PIZOTIFEN, used in the treatment of migraine; the antidepressants AMITRIPTYLINE and FLUPENTHIXOL; the anxiolytic BUSPIRONE; the anti-emetic ONDANSETRON. These illustrate the apparently widespread roles of this interesting mediator.
Related article: HORMONES.

Sevredol (*Napp*) is a proprietary narcotic ANALGESIC on the controlled drugs list. It is used primarily to relieve pain following surgery, or the pain experienced during the final stages of terminal malignant disease. Produced in the form of tablets (in two strengths), it is a preparation of the OPIATE and NARCOTIC morphine sulphate.
▲/ ● side-effects/warning: *see* MORPHINE.

S

Sinemet (*Merck, Sharp & Dohme*) is a proprietary preparation of the powerful drug levodopa in combination with the enyzyme inhibitor CARBIDOPA; it is available only on prescription. Sinemet is used to treat parkinsonism, but not the parkinsonian symptoms induced by drugs (*see* ANTIPARKINSONIAN): the carbidopa prevents too rapid a breakdown of the levodopa (into dopamine) in the periphery, thus allowing more levodopa to reach the brain to make up the deficiency (of dopamine), which is the major cause of parkinsonian symptoms. Sinemet is produced in the form of tablets with a levodopa/carbidopa ratio of 10:1 (in two strengths), and of 4:1 (in two strengths) under the names Sinemet LS and Sinemet Plus.
▲/ ● side-effects/warning: *see* LEVODOPA.

Sinequan (*Pfizer*) is a proprietary ANTIDEPRESSANT drug, available only on prescription. Used especially in cases where sedation is deemed necessary. Produced in the form of capsules (in four strengths), Sinequan is a preparation of the TRICYCLIC antidepressant doxepin. It is not recommended for children.
▲/ ● side-effects/warning: *see* DOXEPIN.

***skeletal muscle relaxants** act on voluntary (skeletal) muscles of the body. Some are used during operations to aid surgery (e.g. tubocurarine) and act by interfering with the actions of the neurotransmitter acetylcholine at sites between nerve and muscle. Others used in the treatment of painful muscle spasms act within the central nervous system (e.g. DIAZEPAM).

Slo-Indo (*Generics*) is a proprietary, ANTI-INFLAMATORY, non-narcotic ANALGESIC (NSAID), available only on prescription, used to relieve the pain of rheumatic disease, gout, and other inflammatory musculo-skeletal disorders. Produced in the form of sustained-release capsules, Slo-Indo is a preparation of indomethacin.
▲/ ● side-effects/warning: *see* INDOMETHACIN.

Sloprolol (*CP Pharmaceuticals*) is a proprietary BETA-BLOCKER available only on prescription. It is used as an ANXIOLYTIC to treat anxiety, and to try to prevent migraine attacks (ANTIMIGRAINE). Produced in the form of sustained-release capsules Sloprolol is a preparation of propranolol hydrochloride.
▲/ ● side-effects/warning: *see* PROPRANOLOL.

Sodium Amytal (*Lilly*) is a proprietary preparation of the BARBITURATE amylobarbitone sodium, a drug on the controlled drugs list, used to relieve intractable insomnia in cases

other than where pain is the cause. Side-effects may be severe – it is not recommended for children – and dependence (addiction) occurs readily. It is produced in the form of capsules (in two strengths) or tablets (in two strengths), or as a powder for reconstitution as a medium for injection.
see AMYLOBARBITONE.

sodium salicylate is a soluble, non-narcotic ANALGESIC and ANTI-INFLAMMATORY (NSAID) agent used in both capacities to treat rheumatic and other musculo-skeletal disorders.
Administration is oral in the form of a non-proprietary mixture (liquid).

▲ side-effects: gastrointestinal upset is common; there may also be nausea, hearing disturbances and vertigo; some patients experience ulceration and bleeding. Rarely, there is a state of confusion, sensitivity reactions (such as asthma-like attacks or a rash), inflammation of the heart, or blood disorders.

✚ warning: sodium salicylate should not be administered to patients with peptic ulcers or who are aged under 12 years; it should be administered with caution to those with severely impaired function of the kidneys or the liver, allergies or dehydration, who are pregnant or lactating, who are elderly, or who are already taking anticoagulant drugs.

sodium valproate is an ANTICONVULSANT drug used to treat epilepsy. It is particularly effective in controlling grand mal (tonic-clonic) seizures in primary generalized epilepsy, although it is used to treat all forms of the disorder. The drug is also occasionally used to treat the rare cases of recurrent febrile convulsions in children, to whom it may be administered prophylactically. Administration is oral in the form of tablets and as a liquid (or dilute syrup).

▲ side-effects: there may be nausea and gastrointestinal disturbance, increased appetite and consequent weight gain, temporary hair loss, and impaired liver function. If severe vomiting and weight loss occur, treatment should be withdrawn at once.

✚ warning: sodium valproate should not be administered to patients with liver disease: liver function should be monitored for at least the first 6 months of treatment. The drug may cause some blood count readings to be misleading in relation to diabetic patients.
Related article: EPILIM.

Solis (*Galen*) is a proprietary ANXIOLYTIC drug, available on prescription only to private patients, used to treat anxiety and insomnia, and to assist in the treatment of acute alcohol withdrawal symptoms. Also a SKELETAL MUSCLE RELAXANT, Solis is sometimes also used to relieve muscle spasm. Produced in the form of capsules (in two strengths), it is a preparation of the BENZODIAZEPINE diazepam. Dependence may result with prolonged use.

▲/✚ side-effects/warning: *see* DIAZEPAM.

Solpadeine (*Sterling Research*) is a proprietary, non-prescription compound ANALGESIC, which is not available from the National Health Service. It is used to relieve the pain of headaches, and of rheumatism and other musculo-skeletal disorders. Produced in the form of tablets for effervescent solution, Solpadeine is a combination of paracetamol,

codeine phosphate and caffeine.
▲/✚ side-effects/warning: *see* CAFFEINE; CODEINE PHOSPHATE; PARACETAMOL.

Solpadol (*Sterling-Winthrop*) is a proprietary compound ANALGESIC, available only on prescription, used as a painkiller particularly for children. Produced in the form of effervescent tablets, Solpadol is a preparation of the OPIATE codeine phosphate and paracetamol, and contains more codeine than the usual compound preparation known as CO-CODAMOL). It is not recommended for children.
▲/✚ side-effects/warning: *see* CODEINE PHOSPHATE; PARACETAMOL.

Solprin (*Reckitt & Colman*) is a proprietary, non-prescription preparation of the non-narcotic ANALGESIC aspirin, which is not available from the National Health Service. It is used to relieve mild to moderate pain, and is produced in the form of soluble (dispersible) tablets.
▲/✚ side-effects/warning: *see* ASPIRIN.

Sominex (*Beecham*) is a proprietary, non-prescription TRANQUILLIZER used to relieve occasional insomnia. Produced in the form of tablets, it is a preparation of the ANTIHISTAMINE promethazine hydrochloride; it is not recommended for children aged under 16 years.
▲/✚ side-effects/warning: *see* PROMETHAZINE HYDROCHLORIDE.

Somnite (*Norgine*) is a proprietary HYPNOTIC, available on prescription only to private patients, used in the short term to treat insomnia in patients for whom daytime sedation is not appropriate. Produced in the form of a suspension (for swallowing), Somnite is a preparation of the BENZODIAZEPINE nitrazepam. Dependence may result with prolonged use. It is not recommended for children.
▲/✚ side-effects/warning: *see* NITRAZEPAM.

Soneryl (*May & Baker*) is a proprietary sedative, a BARBITURATE on the controlled drugs list, used as a HYPNOTIC to treat intractable insomnia. Produced in the form of tablets, it is a preparation of butobarbitone. It is not recommended for children or the elderly.
▲/✚ side-effects/warning: *see* BUTOBARBITONE.

Sparine (*Wyeth*) is a proprietary ANTIPSYCHOTIC drug, available only on prescription, used to soothe agitation (particularly in the elderly or the dying) and for the short-term relief of acute, severe anxiety. It is also sometimes used to calm children prior to cardiac investigation or electro-encephalography. Produced in the form of tablets (in three strengths), as a suspension for dilution (the potency of the suspension once dilute is retained for 14 days) and in ampoules for injection, Sparine is a preparation of promazine hydrochloride. It is not recommended for children other than for the purpose outlined above.
▲/✚ side-effects/warning: *see* PROMAZINE HYDROCHLORIDE.

Stelazine (*Smith, Kline & French*) is a proprietary form of the ANTIPSYCHOTIC drug trifluoperazine. Available only on prescription, it is used to treat psychoses (such as schizophrenia) including the control of behavioural disturbances. It may be used alternatively to treat anxiety in the short-term and as an ANTI-EMETIC for nausea and

vomiting. Stelazine is produced in the form of tablets (in two strengths), as sustained-release capsules (spansules, in three strengths), as a sugar-free syrup for dilution, and in ampoules for injection.
▲/ ● side-effects/warning: *see* TRIFLUOPERAZINE.

Stemetil (*May & Baker*) is a proprietary ANTI-EMETIC, available only on prescription, used to relieve symptoms of nausea caused by the vertigo and loss of balance experienced in disorders of the inner and middle ears, or by cytotoxic drugs in the treatment of cancer. Produced in the form of tablets (in two strengths), as a syrup for dilution (the potency of the syrup once dilute is retained for 14 days), as anal suppositories (in two strengths), and in ampoules for injection, Stemetil is a preparation of the major TRANQUILLIZER prochlorperazine.
▲/ ● side-effects/warning: *see* PROCHLORPERAZINE.

Stesolid (*CP Pharmaceuticals*) is a proprietary ANXIOLYTIC drug, available only on prescription, used to treat anxiety and insomnia, to act as a premedication before surgery, and to assist in the treatment of acute alcohol withdrawal symptoms. Also a SKELETAL MUSCLE RELAXANT and an ANTICONVULSANT, Stesolid is used to treat muscle spasm and – more seriously – convulsions due to poisoning and to epileptic seizures. Produced in the form of tubes (for rectal insertion), Stesolid is a preparation of the potentially addictive BENZODIAZEPINE diazepam. It is not recommended for children aged under 12 months.
▲/ ● side-effects/warning: *see* DIAZEPAM.

***stimulants** are agents that activate body systems or functions. In general, the term is applied to drugs that stimulate the central nervous system. The result may be increased attention or mental energy, wakefulness, increased enthusiasm, and perhaps mild euphoria, but such effects are only temporary and the return to ordinary actuality may leave the individual physically tired and more 'down' than before. Chronic, high doses of amphetamine-like stimulants can lead to sleep deprivation and a psychotic state. Yet patients who suffer from nacrolepsy (a sleep-like state), and children who are hyperactive may well derive some therapeutic benefit from the administration of certain types of stimulant. Although their use in children must be carefully supervised. Central nervous system stimulants include the amphetamines (such as DEXAMPHETAMINE SULPHATE) and CAFFEINE (found in tea and coffee). Cocaine may be classed as a central nervous system stimulant.

Stugeron (*Janssen*) is a proprietary, non-prescription preparation of the ANTIHISTAMINE cinnarizine, used to treat nausea caused by the vertigo and loss of balance experienced in infections of the middle and inner ears. It is produced in the form of tablets.
▲/ ● side-effects/warning: *see* CINNARIZINE.

Sublimaze (*Janssen*) is a narcotic ANALGESIC on the controlled drugs list, primarily used to enhance the effect of a BARBITURATE general ANAESTHETIC, allowing the barbiturate dose to be smaller. Produced in ampoules for injection, Sublimaze is a

S

preparation of the morphine-like drug fentanyl.
▲/ ● side-effects/warning: *see* FENTANYL.

sulindac is a non-steroidal, ANTI-INFLAMMATORY, non-narcotic ANALGESIC (NSAID) drug used to treat pain and inflammation in rheumatic disease and other musculo-skeletal disorders, and acute gout. Administration is by tablets.
▲ side-effects: there may be nausea and gastrointestinal disturbance; internal haemorrhage may occur. Some patients experience sensitivity reactions such as a rash, headache, asthma-like symptoms, and even vertigo or ringing in the ears (tinnitus). Rarely, there is fluid retention leading to weight gain, or a minor change in the composition of the blood.
● warning: sulindac should be administered with caution to patients with impaired liver or kidney function, gastric ulcers, allergic conditions, or who are pregnant, or have a history of renal stones. Adequate hydration should be maintained.
Related article: CLINORIL.

sulpiride is an atypical benzamide ANTIPSYCHOTIC drug, with some ANTIDEPRESSANT properties, used to treat the symptoms of schizophrenia. In low doses, it increases an apathetic, withdrawn patient's awareness and tends to generate a true consciousness of events. In high doses it is also used to treat other conditions that may cause tremor, tics, involuntary movements or involuntary utterances (such as the relatively uncommon Gilles de la Tourette syndrome). Administration is oral in the form of tablets.
▲ side-effects: extrapyramidal motor disorders seem to be less likely to occur than with other antipsychotics. There may be restlessness, agitation and insomnia.
● warning: sulpiride should not be administered to patients with tumour of adrenal chromaffin tissue (phaeochromocytoma), porphyria, or who are breast-feeding. Experience of the drugs effects in children is limited.
Related articles: DOLMATIL; SULPITIL.

Sulpitil (*Tillotts*) is a proprietary ANTIPSYCHOTIC drug used to treat the symptoms of schizophrenia. In low doses, it increases an apathetic, withdrawn patient's awareness and tends to generate a true consciousness of events. In high doses it is also used to treat other conditions that may cause tremor, tics, involuntary movements or involuntary utterances (such as the relatively uncommon Gilles de la Tourette syndrome). Produced in the form of tablets, Sulpitil is a preparation of sulpiride. It is not recommended for children under the age of 14.
▲/ ● side-effects/warning: *see* SULPIRIDE.

Surem (*Galen*) is a proprietary HYPNOTIC, available on prescription only to private patients, used in the short-term to treat insomnia in patients for whom daytime sedation is not appropriate. Produced in the form of capsules, Surem is a preparation of the BENZODIAZEPINE nitrazepam. It is not recommended for children. Dependence may result with prolonged use.
▲/ ● side-effects/warning: *see* NITRAZEPAM.

Surgam (*Roussel*) is a proprietary, non-narcotic, ANALGESIC, available only on prescription, used to treat the pain of rheumatic disease and other musculo-

S

skeletal disorders. Produced in the form of tablets (in two strengths, under the names Surgam 200 and Surgam 300), it is a preparation of the non-steroidal, ANTI-INFLAMMATORY (NSAID) agent tiaprofenic acid.
▲/ ✚ side-effects/warning: *see* TIAPROFENIC ACID.

Surmontil (*Rorer*) is a proprietary ANTIDEPRESSANT, available only on prescription, used to treat depressive illness (especially in cases where there is a need for sedation), and severe insomnia. Produced in the form of tablets (in two strengths) and as capsules, Surmontil is a preparation of the TRICYCLIC drug trimipramine maleate. It is not recommended for children.
▲/ ✚ side-effects/warning: *see* TRIMIPRAMINE.

Symmetrel (*Geigy*) is a proprietary preparation of the powerful drug amantadine hydrochloride, available only on prescription, used to treat parkinsonism, but not the parkinsonian symptoms induced by drugs (*see* ANTIPARKINSONIAN). Effective on some patients, but not on others, Symmetrel is produced in the form of capsules and as a syrup for dilution (the potency of the syrup once dilute is retained for 4 weeks).
▲/ ✚ side-effects/warning: *see* AMANTADINE HYDROCHLORIDE.

***sympathomimetics** are drugs that have effects mimicking those of the sympathetic nervous system. There are two main types, although several sympathomimetics belong to both types. Alpha-adrenergic sympathomimetics (such as phenylephrine) are VASOCONSTRICTORS and are particularly used in nasal decongestants. Beta-adrenergic sympathomimetics (such as salbutamol) are frequently smooth muscle relaxants, particularly on bronchial smooth muscle, and are used especially as bronchodilators.
see NORADRENALINE;

Synflex (*Syntex*) is a proprietary, non-narcotic ANALGESIC, available only on prescription, used to treat migraine (*see* ANTIMIGRAINE) and menstrual and inflammatory pain, and pain following surgery. Produced in the form of tablets, it is a preparation of the non- steroidal ANTI-INFLAMMATORY drug naproxen sodium.
▲/ ✚ side-effects/warning: *see* NAPROXEN.

Tancolin (*Ashe*) is a proprietary, non-prescription ANTITUSSIVE, which is not available from the National Health Service. Orange-flavoured, its active constituents include the bronchodilator theophylline, the NARCOTIC cough suppressant dextromethorphan, the antacid sodium citrate, and ascorbic acid (vitamin C).
▲/✚ side-effects/warning: *see* DEXTROMETHORPHAN.

Teejel (*Napp*) is a proprietary, non-prescription gel containing both an antiseptic and an ANALGESIC, used to treat mouth ulcers, sore gums or inflammation of the tongue. The gel is intended to be massaged in gently. It consists of a compound of the analgesic choline salicylate with the antiseptic cetalkonium chloride (both in solution). It is not recommended for children aged under 4 months.
▲/✚ side-effects/warning: *see* CHOLINE SALICYLATE.

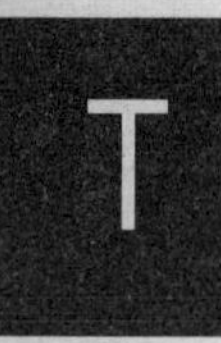

Tegretol (*Geigy*) is a proprietary preparation of the ANTICONVULSANT drug carbamazapine, available only on prescription, used to treat several forms of epilepsy, including generalized tonic-clonic and partial seizures, and to relieve trigeminal neuralgia (pain in the side of the face). It also has applications in the treatment of manic-depressive illness. Tegretol may also be beneficial in the treatment of aspects of diabetes and diabetes insipidus. It is produced in the form of tablets (in three strengths), chewable tablets (in two strengths), as a sugar-free liquid for dilution (the potency of the liquid once dilute is retained for 14 days), and as controlled-release tablets under the trade name Tegretol Retard (in two strengths).
▲/✚ side-effects/warning: *see* CARBAMAZEPINE.

temazepam is a relatively short-acting BENZODIAZEPINES, used as a TRANQUILLIZER to treat insomnia (particularly in the elderly) and as an ANXIOLYTIC premedication prior to surgery. Administration is oral in the form of capsules, which are hard or gel-filled (some known as Gelthix), or as an oral solution.
▲ side-effects: concentration and speed of reaction are affected. There may also be drowsiness and unsteadiness. Some patients experience sensitivity reactions. It should be used for short-term treatment only because prolonged use may eventually result in tolerance, and finally dependence.
✚ warning: temazepam should be administered with caution to patients with lung disease or shallow breathing, or impaired liver or kidney function, who are pregnant or lactating, or who are elderly and debilitated.

Temgesic (*Reckitt & Colman*) is a proprietary narcotic ANALGESIC, available only on prescription, used to treat moderate to severe pain. Produced in the form of tablets to be retained under the tongue, and in ampoules for injection, it is a preparation of the OPIATE buprenorphine hydrochloride.
▲/✚ side-effects/warning: *see* BUPRENORPHINE.

tenoxicam is a non-steroidal, ANTI-INFLAMMATORY, non-narcotic ANALGESIC (NSAID) drug. It is used to treat rheumatic and muscular pain caused by inflammation and/or bone degeneration particularly at the joints.
▲ side-effects: relatively uncommon, but gastrointestinal disturbances with nausea may occur and patients may be advise to take

the drug with food or milk. There may be sensitivity reactions.

⬢ warning: tenoxicam should be adminstered with caution to patients with allergic disorders, impaired liver or kidney function, gastric ulcers, or who are pregnant.
Related article: MOBIFLEX.

Tensium (*DDSA Pharmaceuticals*) is a proprietary ANXIOLYTIC drug, available on prescription only to private patients. It is used for short-term treatment of insomnia and anxiety, and to relieve the effects of acute alcohol withdrawal symptoms. Produced in the form of tablets (in three strengths), Tensium is a preparation of the powerful and long-acting BENZODIAZEPINE diazepam. Prolonged use may result in dependence.

▲/⬢ side-effects/warning: *see* DIAZEPAM.

Tenuate Dospan (*Merrell*) is a proprietary preparation of the amphetamine-related drug diethylpropion hydrochloride, used as an APPETITE SUPPRESSANT in the medical treatment of obesity. On the controlled drugs list, it is produced in the form of sustained-release tablets. Treatment must be in the short term and under strict medical supervision.

▲/⬢ side-effects/warning: *see* DIETHYLPROPION HYDROCHLORIDE.

Tercoda (*Sinclair*) is a proprietary, non-prescription cough elixir that is not available from the National Health Service. It's active constituents include codeine phosphate and the EXPECTORANT terpin hydrate.

▲/⬢ side-effects/warning: *see* CODEINE PHOSPHATE.

Teronac (*Sandoz*) is a proprietary preparation of the stimulant drug mazindol, used as an APPETITE-SUPPRESSANT in the medical treatment of obesity. On the controlled drugs list (because it is potentially addictive and anorective), it is produced in the form of tablets. Treatment must be in the short term and under strict medical supervision.

▲/⬢ side-effects/warning: *see* MAZINDOL.

Terpoin (*Hough*) is a proprietary ANTITUSSIVE cough elixir, available on prescription only to private patients. Active constituents include codeine phosphate, the expectorant guaiphenesin, and menthol.

▲/⬢ side-effects/warning: *see* CODEINE PHOSPHATE.

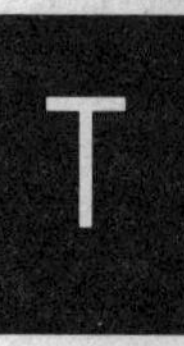

tetrabenazine is a powerful drug used to assist a patient to regain voluntary control of movement – or at least to lessen the extent of involuntary movements – in Huntington's chorea and related disorders. It is thought to work by reducing the amount of DOPAMINE in the nerve endings in the brain. Administration is oral in the form of tablets.

▲ side-effects: there may be drowsiness and postural hypotension. Some patients experience depression.

⬢ warning: tetrabenazine should not be administered to patients who are lactating or who are already taking drugs that contain levodopa or reserpine.
Related article: NITOMAN.

Thalamonal (*Janssen*) is a proprietary preparation of the TRANQUILLIZER droperidol and the narcotic ANALGESIC fentanyl, and is accordingly on the controlled drugs list. It is used on patients about to undergo diagnostic or minor surgical procedures that may be difficult or painful. It is produced in ampoules for injection.

▲/♣ side-effects/warning: *see* DROPERIDOL; FENTANYL.

thiethylperazine is an ANTI-EMETIC drug used to relieve nausea and vomiting that may be caused by the vertigo associated with disorders of the inner or middle ear, or by therapy with cytotoxic drugs in the treatment of cancer. Administration is oral in the form of tablets, topical as anal suppositories, or by injection.

▲ side-effects: there is commonly drowsiness; there may also be dry mouth and dizziness on rising from sitting or lying down (caused by low blood pressure). Some patients, particularly young women, experience muscle spasms.

♣ warning: thiethylperazine should not be administered to patients who are in a coma, or have glaucoma or impaired capacity of the bone-marrow to produce blood cells. It should be administered with caution to those with heart or lung disease, dysfunction of the adrenal glands in the secretion of hormones, epilepsy, parkinsonism, impaired kidney or liver function, undersecretion of thyroid hormones, or enlargement of the prostate gland. Regular ophthalmic checks and monitoring of skin pigmentation are required. Treatment should be withdrawn gradually.
Related article: TORECAN.

thiopentone sodium is a widely used general ANAESTHETIC used during operations. It has no analgesic properties. Because the drug is exceptionally powerful, however, inadvertent overdosage does occur from time to time, causing respiratory depression and depression of the heart rate. Both initial induction of anaesthesia and awakening afterwards are smooth and rapid, although some sedative effects may endure for up to 24 hours. Administration is by injection.

▲ side-effects: there may be respiratory depression, and means for treating respiratory failure should be available. During induction with thiopentone sodium, sneezing, coughing and bronchial spasm may occur.

♣ warning: thiopentone sodium should not be given to patients whose respiratory tract is obstructed, those in severe shock, or those with porphyria (poor porphyrin metabolism). Caution should be taken when administering the drug to patients with severe liver or kidney disease, with metabolic disorders, or who are elderly.

thioridazine is a phenothiazine ANTIPSYCHOTIC drug used to treat psychosis (such as schizophrenia), in which it is particularly suitable for treating manic forms of behavioural disturbance, especially in order to effect emergency control. The drug may also be used to treat anxiety in the short-term and to calm agitated elderly patients. It is less likely than other antipsychotics to cause extrapyramidal motor disorders, and is therefore suitable for elderly patients. However, it is more likely to lower blood pressure. Administration is oral in the form of tablets or a liquid.

▲ side-effects: concentration and speed of thought and movement are affected. Rashes and jaundice may occur; and there may be dry mouth, gastrointestinal disturbance, difficulties in urinating, male sexual dysfunction, a reduction in blood pressure, and blurred or discoloured vision.

♦ warning: thioridazine should not be administered to patients who suffer from a reduction in the bone-marrow's capacity to produce blood cells, or from certain types of glaucoma, or porphyria. It should be administered only with caution to those with heart or vascular disease, kidney or liver disease, parkinsonism, or depression; or who are pregnant or lactating. It is not recommended for children.
Related article: MELLERIL.

tiaprofenic acid is a non-steroidal, ANTI-INFLAMMATORY, non-narcotic ANALGESIC (NSAID) used to treat pain and inflammation in rheumatic disease and other musculo-skeletal disorders. Administration is oral in the form of tablets or an infusion.
▲ side-effects: there may be nausea and gastrointestinal disturbance (to avoid which a patient may be advised to take the drug with food or milk), headache and ringing in the ears (tinnitus). Some patients experience sensitivity reactions (such as the symptoms of asthma). Fluid retention and/or blood disorders may occur.
♦ warning: tiaprofenic acid should be administered with caution to patients with gastric ulcers, impaired kidney or liver function, or allergic disorders, or who are pregnant.
Related article: SURGAM.

timolol maleate is a BETA-BLOCKER used as an ANTIMIGRAINE to treat and prevent migraine attacks. Administration is thus oral in the form of tablets or capsules.
▲ side-effects: there may be gastrointestinal disturbances, slow heart rate and cold fingertips and toes, and symptoms much like asthma.
♦ warning: timolol maleate should not be administered to patients with asthma, bradycardia (slow heartbeat) or partial heart block; it should be administered with caution to those with congestive heart failure, impaired liver or kidney function, who are diabetic, or who are pregnant or lactating. Withdrawal of treatment should be gradual.
Related article: BETIM.

Tixylix (*May & Baker*) is a proprietary, non-prescription compound cough linctus, which is not available from the National Health Service. Produced in the form of a syrup for dilution (the potency of the syrup once dilute is retained for 14 days), Tixylix is a preparation of the opiate ANTITUSSIVE pholcodine citrate and the ANTIHISTAMINE promethazine hydrochloride.
▲/♦ side-effects/warning: *see* PHOLCODINE; PROMETHAZINE HYDROCHLORIDE.

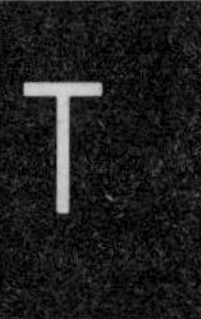

Tofranil (*Geigy*) is a proprietary TRICYCLIC ANTIDEPRESSANT drug, available only on prescription, used to treat depressive illness particularly in patients who are withdrawn and apathetic. It may also be used to treat nocturnal bedwetting by children (aged over 7 years). Produced in the form of tablets (in two strengths) and as a syrup for dilution (the potency of the syrup once diluted is retained for 14 days), Tofranil is a preparation of imipramine hydrochloride. Treatment may be prolonged.
▲/♦ side-effects/warning: *see* IMIPRAMINE.

Tolectin (*Ortho-Cilag*) is a proprietary preparation of the non-steroidal drug tolmetrin, which has ANTI-INFLAMMATORY, non-narcotic ANALGESIC (NSAID) properties. Available only on

prescription, it is used to treat the pain of rheumatic disease and other musculo-skeletal disorders (including bone fusion). It is produced in the form of capsules in two strengths.
▲/● side-effects/warning: *see* TOLMETIN.

tolmetin is a non-steroidal drug with ANTI-INFLAMMATORY (NSAID) and ANALGESIC properties used to treat the pain of rheumatic disease and other musculo-skeletal disorders. Administration is oral in the form of capsules.
▲ side-effects: there may be nausea and gastrointestinal disturbance (to avoid which a patient might be advised to take the drug with food or milk), headache and ringing in the ears (tinnitus). Some patients experience sensitivity reactions (such as the symptoms of asthma). Fluid retention and/or blood disorders may occur.
● warning: tolmetin should be administered with caution to patients with gastric ulcers, impaired kidney or liver function, bleeding disorders, cardio-vascular disease or allergic disorders, or who are pregnant.
Related article: TOLECTIN.

Torecan (*Sandoz*) is a proprietary ANTI-EMETIC drug, available only on prescription, used to relieve nausea and vomiting that may be caused by the vertigo associated with disorders of the middle or inner ear, or by therapy with cytotoxic drugs in the treatment of cancer. Produced in the form of tablets, as anal suppositories, and in ampoules for injection, Torecan is a preparation of thiethylperazine.
▲/● side-effects/warning: *see* THIETHYLPERAZINE.

Trancopal (*Winthrop*) is a proprietary ANXIOLYTIC drug that also has the properties of a SKELETAL MUSCLE RELAXANT. Available only on prescription, it is used principally in the short-term treatment of insomnia, and produced in the form of tablets containing the TRANQUILLIZER chlormezanone. It is not recommended for children.
▲/● side-effects/warning: *see* CHLORMEZANONE.

***tranquillizers** are drugs that calm and soothe, and relieve anxiety. Many also cause some degree of sedation. They are classified into two very different groups, major and minor tranquillizers. The major tranquillizers, also called NEUROLEPTICS or ANTIPSYCHOTIC agents, are used primarily to treat severe mental disorders where the processes of thought and reasoning are distorted – the psychoses (including schizophrenia). In this situation they are highly effective in restoring a patient to a calmer, less disturbed state of mind. The hallucinations, both auditory and visual, the gross disturbance of logical thinking and to some extent the delusions typical of psychotic states are generally well controlled by these drugs. Violent, aggressive behaviour that presents a danger to the patients themselves and to those who look after them is also effectively treated by major tranquillizers. For this reason they are also often used in the 'management' of difficult, aggressive, anti-social individuals. Widely prescribed major tranquillizers include the PHENOTHIAZINES (such as CHLORPROMAZINE, THIORIDAZINE and PROCHLORPERAZINE) and such drugs as HALOPERIDOL, FLUSPIRILENE and FLUPENTHIXOL.

Minor tranquillizers are also 'calming' drugs, but they are ineffective in the treatment of psychotic states. Their principal applications are as hypnotic, sedative and ANXIOLYTIC drugs. The best-known and most widely prescribed minor tranquillizers are undoubtedly the BENZODIAZEPINES (such as DIAZEPAM and CHLORDIAZEPOXIDE). Prolonged treatment with minor tranquillizers can lead to dependence (addiction).

Tranxene (*Boehringer Ingelheim*) is a proprietary ANXIOLYTIC drug, available only on prescription to private patients, used principally in the short-term treatment of anxiety. Produced in the form of capsules (in two strengths), it is a preparation of the TRANQUILLIZER clorazepate dipotassium. It is not recommended for children and it may cause dependence.

▲/ ✚ side-effects/warning: *see* CLORAZEPATE DIPOTASSIUM.

tranylcypromine is an ANTIDEPRESSANT drug, a MAO INHIBITOR that also has some stimulant effect and is therefore less used than most in the treatment of depressive illness. Administration is oral in the form of tablets.

▲ side-effects: concentration and speed of thought and movement are usually affected; there may also be dizziness, especially when rising from sitting or lying down (because of low blood pressure), and insomnia, muscular weakness and dry mouth. Some patients experience severe headache, which implies that treatment should be withdrawn. Some patients experience insomnia if the drug is taken in the evening.

✚ warning: tranylcypromine should not be administered to patients with heart or liver disease, circulatory disorders, abnormal secretion of hormones by the adrenal glands, epilepsy, or overactivity of the thyroid gland (hyperthyroidism), or who are children. It should be administered with caution to those who are elderly or debilitated. Treatment requires a strict dietary regime (that includes the avoidance of meat or yeast extracts, cheese, and alcohol) and the avoidance also of virtually all other forms of medication. Withdrawal of treatment must be gradual.

Related article: PARNATE; PARSTELIN.

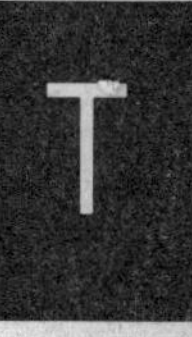

trazodone hydrochloride is an ANTIDEPRESSANT drug used to treat depressive illness, particularly in cases where some degree of sedation is called for. Administration is oral in the form of capsules or a liquid.

▲ side-effects: common effects include sedation (affecting driving ability), dry mouth and blurred vision; there may also be difficulty in urinating, sweating and irregular heartbeat, behavioural disturbances, a rash, a state of confusion, and/or a loss of libido. Rarely, there are also blood disorders.

✚ warning: trazodone hydrochloride should not be administered to patients who suffer from heart disease or psychosis; it should be administered with caution to patients who suffer from diabetes, epilepsy, liver or thyroid disease, glaucoma or urinary retention; or who are pregnant or lactating. Withdrawal of treatment must be gradual.

Related article: MOLIPAXIN.

Tremonil (*Sandoz*) is a proprietary drug used to treat the tremor of parkinsonism, of drug-induced states, or simply of old age (*see* ANTIPARKINSONIAN). Available only on prescription, and produced in the form of tablets, it is a preparation of methixene hydrochloride.
▲/✚ side-effects/warning: *see* METHIXENE HYDROCHLORIDE.

triclofos sodium is a derivative of the soluble SEDATIVE chloral, used as a HYPNOTIC in the short-term to treat insomnia. Administration is oral in the form of an elixir: the liquid is less irritant to the stomach lining than chloral hydrate.
▲ side-effects: concentration and speed of thought and movement are affected. There is commonly drowsiness, dry mouth and gastric irritation; there may also be sensitivity reactions (such as a rash) and, in the elderly, a mild state of confusion.
✚ warning: triclofos sodium should not be administered to patients with severe heart disease, or severe impairment of kidney or liver function. It should be administered with caution to those with lung disease, particularly if there is depressed breathing, who are elderly or debilitated, or who are pregnant or lactating. The consumption of alcohol enhances the hypnotic effect of the drug. Withdrawal of treatment should be gradual. Prolonged use may lead to tolerance and dependence (addiction).

***tricyclic** drugs are one of the two main classes of ANTIDEPRESSANT, and often have SEDATIVE and TRANQUILLIZER effects. Chemically, they are dibenzazipine or debenzocycloheptone derivatives. Examples include AMITRIPTYLINE and LOFEPRAMINE.

trifluoperazine is a phenothiazine ANTIPSYCHOTIC drug used to treat psychosis (such as schizophrenia), and severe forms of behavioural disturbance. The drug may additionally be used to treat severe anxiety in the short term. In low dosages the drug is also sometimes used as an ANTI-EMETIC in the treatment of nausea and vomiting caused by underlying disease or by drug therapies. Trifluoperazine is less sedating, but more likely to cause extrapyramidal motor disorders than some other antipsychotics. Administration is oral in the form of tablets, capsules, sustained-release capsules, and a liquid, or by injection.
▲ side-effects: extrapyramidal motor disorders may occur (muscle spasms, restlessness, tremor) and, with prolonged high dosage, tardive dyskinesias. Concentration and speed of thought and movement are affected. There may be restlessness, insomnia and nightmares; rashes and jaundice may occur; and there may be dry mouth, slight gastrointestinal disturbance, and blurred vision. Some patients experience muscle weakness.
✚ warning: trifluoperazine should not be administered to patients who suffer from reduction in the bone-marrow's capacity to produce blood cells, or from certain types of glaucoma. It should be administered only with caution to those with heart or vascular disease, kidney or liver disease, or parkinsonism; or who are pregnant or lactating.
Related article: PARSTELIN; STELAZINE.

T

trifluperidol is a butyrophenone ANTIPSYCHOTIC drug used to treat psychoses (such as schizophrenia), and forms of manic behavioural disturbance. It is less sedating, but more likely to cause extrapyramidal motor disorders than some of the antipsychotics. Administration is oral in the form of tablets.

▲ side-effects: extrapyramidal motor disorders may occur (muscle spasms, restlessness, tremor) and, with prolonged high dosage, tardive dyskinesias. Concentration and speed of thought and movement are affected.

● warning: trifluperidol should not be administered to patients who suffer from reduction in the bone-marrow's capacity to produce blood cells, or those with excessive thyroid secretion. It should be administered only with caution to those with heart or vascular disease, kidney or liver disease, or parkinsonism, or who are pregnant or lactating, or depressed.

Related article: TRIPERIDOL.

Trilisate (*Napp*) is a proprietary, non-prescription, non-narcotic, ANTI-INFLAMMATORY ANALGESIC used to treat pain and inflammation in rheumatic disease and other musculoskeletal disorders. Produced in the form of tablets, it is a compound preparation of choline and SALICYLIC ACID.

▲/● side-effects/warning: *see* CHOLINE MAGNESIUM TRISALICYLATE.

trimeprazine tartrate is an ANTIHISTAMINE that has additional SEDATIVE properties. It is used as a premedication prior to surgery, and sometimes as an ANTI-EMETIC. Administration is oral in the form of tablets or as a dilute syrup.

▲ side-effects: there may be headache, drowsiness and dry mouth. Some patients experience sensitivity reactions on the skin.

● warning: trimeprazine tartrate should be administered with caution to patients with epilepsy, glaucoma, liver disease or enlargement of the prostate gland. During treatment, alcohol consumption must be avoided.

trimipramine is a TRICYCLIC ANTIDEPRESSANT drug used to treat depressive illness, especially in cases where sedation is advantageous to the patient. Administration of trimipramine is oral in the form of capsules or tablets.

▲ side-effects: common effects include sedation (affecting driving ability), dry mouth and blurred vision; there may also be difficulty in urinating, sweating and irregular heartbeat, behavioural disturbances, a rash, a state of confusion, and/or a loss of libido. Rarely, there are also blood disorders.

● warning: trimipramine should not be administered to patients who suffer from heart disease or psychosis; it should be administered with caution to patients who suffer from diabetes, epilepsy, liver or thyroid disease, glaucoma or urinary retention; or who are pregnant or lactating. Withdrawal of treatment must be gradual.

Related article: SURMONTIL.

Triperidol (*Lagap*) is a proprietary ANTIPSYCHOTIC drug, available only on prescription, used to treat psychosis (such as schizophrenia), and forms of manic behavioural disturbance. Produced in the form of tablets (in two strengths),

Triperidol is a preparation of trifluperidol.
▲/ ⬣ side-effects/warning: *see* TRIFLUPERIDOL.

Triptafen (*Allen & Hanburys*) is a proprietary compound ANTIDEPRESSANT, available only on prescription, used to treat depressive illness particularly in cases in which there is also anxiety. Produced in the form of tablets (in two strengths, the weaker under the name Triptafen-M), it is a combination of amitriptyline hydrochloride with the PHENOTHIAZINE antipsychotic perphenazine. It is not recommended for children.
▲/ ⬣ side-effects/warning: *see* AMITRIPTYLINE; PERPHENAZINE.

T

Tropium (*DDSA Pharmaceuticals*) is a proprietary ANXIOLYTIC drug, available on prescription only to private patients, used to treat anxiety or to assist in the treatment of acute alcohol withdrawal symptoms. Produced in the form of capsules (in two strengths) and tablets (in three strengths), Tropium is a preparation of the BENZODIAZEPINE chlordiazepoxide. Prolonged use may result in dependence.
▲/ ⬣ side-effects/warning: *see* CHLORDIAZEPOXIDE.

Tryptizol (*Morson*) is a proprietary, TRICYCLIC ANTIDEPRESSANT drug, available only on prescription, used in the treatment of depressive illness and especially in cases where its additional SEDATIVE properties may be advantageous to the patients or to those that care for them. However, the drug is additionally used to prevent bedwetting at night in youngsters. Produced in the form of tablets (in three strengths), as sustained-release capsules, as a sugar-free liquid for dilution (the potency of the liquid once dilute is retained for 14 days), and in vials for injection, Tryptizol is a preparation of amitryptyline hydrochloride.
▲/ ⬣ side-effects/warning: *see* AMITRIPTYLINE.

tryptophan is an amino acid present in an ordinary diet, from which the natural body substance SEROTONIN (5-hydroxytryptamine) is derived. Therapeutic administration of tryptophan, singly or in combination with ANTIDEPRESSANTS, has been found to be helpful in certain cases of depressive illness. The response to treatment with tryptophan alone is slow, taking at least 4 weeks for genuine improvement to occur. It is now rarely used. Administration is oral in the form of tablets.
▲ side-effects: concentration and speed of thought and movement may initially be affected; with drowsiness, there may also be nausea and/or a headache.
⬣ warning: tryptophan should not be administered to patients known to have defective metabolism of tryptophan in the diet, or who have disease of the bladder, or who are being treated with the serotonin uptake inhibitors FLUVOXAMINE or FLUOXETINE.

Tuinal (*Lilly*) is a proprietary HYPNOTIC, a BARBITURATE on the controlled drugs list, and used to treat intractable insomnia. Produced in the form of capsules, it is a preparation of amylobarbitone sodium. It is not recommended for children.
▲/ ⬣ side-effects/warning: *see* AMYLOBARBITONE.

Tylex (*Cilag*) is a proprietary compound ANALGESIC, available only on prescription, used as a painkiller. Produced in the form of tablets, Tylex is a preparation of the OPIATE codeine phosphate and paracetamol in the ratio 30:500 (mg), and therefore contains more codeine than the usual compound preparation known as CO-CODAMOL). It is not recommended for children.

▲/ ● side-effects/warning: *see* CODEINE PHOSPHATE; PARACETAMOL.

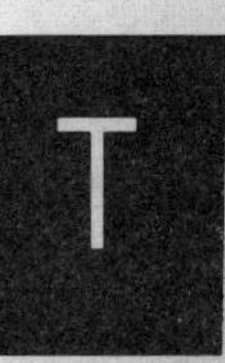

Uniflu Plus Gregovite C (*Unigreg*) is a proprietary combination of two drugs issued as separate tablets to be taken simultaneously to treat the symptoms of colds and influenza. Uniflu is an ANTITUSSIVE and ANTIHISTAMINE that also has some ANALGESIC properties. Because Uniflu contains the OPIATE codeine, however, the combination is not available on a National Health Service prescription; other principal constituents of Uniflu include paracetamol and caffeine. Gregovite C is a form of ASCORBIC ACID (vitamin C).
▲/ ✚ side-effects/warning: *see* CAFFEINE; CODEINE PHOSPHATE; PARACETAMOL.

Unigesic (*Unimed*) is a proprietary compound ANALGESIC not available on a National Health Service prescription, which principally consists of a mixture of paracetamol and caffeine.
▲/ ✚ side-effects/warning: *see* CAFFEINE; PARACETAMOL.

Unisomnia (*Unigreg*) is a proprietary form of the BENZODIAZEPINE nitrazepam. A powerful and long-acting HYPNOTIC produced in the form of tablets, Unisomnia is available only by prescription for private patients. Prolonged use may result in dependence.
▲/ ✚ side-effects/warning: *see* NITRAZEPAM.

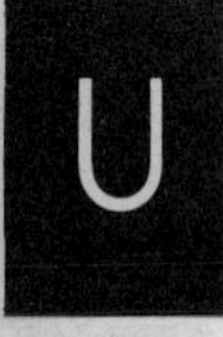

Valenac (*Shire*) is a proprietary form of the non-steroidal, ANTI-INFLAMMATORY (NSAID) drug diclofenac sodium. Available on prescription only as tablets (in two strengths) to treat pain and inflammation of musculo-skeletal disorders, such as rheumatic disease.
▲/✚ side-effects/warning: *see* DICLOFENAC SODIUM.

Valium (*Roche*) is a proprietary form of the powerful BENZODIAZEPINE diazepam, useful as an ANXIOLYTIC or minor TRANQUILLIZER, as a SKELETAL MUSCLE RELAXANT, and also as an ANTICONVULSANT in the treatment of status epilepticus and convulsions due to poisoning. Available only on prescription, it is produced as anal suppositories and in ampoules for injection (available on National Health Service prescription), and as tablets and syrup (available only to private patients). It is prescribed mainly to treat anxiety.
▲/✚ side-effects/warning: *see* DIAZEPAM.

Valoid (*Calmic*) is a proprietary form of ANTIHISTAMINE prescribed as an ANTI-EMETIC to treat vomiting, motion sickness and loss of the sense of balance (labyrinthitis). It comes in two forms: tablets, containing cyclizine hydrochloride and available without prescription; and ampoules for injection, containing cyclizine lactate and available only on prescription.
▲/✚ side-effects/warning: *see* ANTIHISTAMINE; CYCLIZINE.

Valrox (*Cox, CP Pharmaceuticals Ltd*) is a proprietary form of the non-steroidal, ANTI-INFLAMMATORY (NSAID), non-narcotic ANALGESIC drug naproxen. Available on prescription only, it is used to treat pain and inflammation associated with rheumatic disease and other musculo-skeletal disorders. Administered in the form of tablets (in two strengths).
▲/✚ side-effects/warning: *see* NAPROXEN.

***vasoconstrictors** cause a narrowing of the blood vessels, and thus a reduction in the rate of blood flow and an increase in blood pressure. They are used to increase blood pressure in circulatory disorders, in cases of shock, or in cases where pressure has fallen during lengthy or complex surgery.

***vasodilators** cause a widening of the blood vessels, causing changes in blood flow and a reduction in blood pressure. They are used to reduce blood pressure mainly in the treatment of heart failure or angina pectoris (heart pain), to improve the circulation in the brain or in the limbs, or simply to treat high blood pressure (hypertension).
Related articles: CYCLANDELATE; CYCLOSPASMOL.

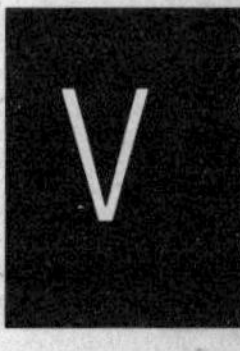

Veganin (*Warner*) is a proprietary, non-prescription compound ANALGESIC, which is not available from the National Health Service, consisting of tablets that contain aspirin, codeine phosphate and paracetamol.
▲/✚ side-effects/warning: *see* ASPIRIN; CODEINE PHOSPHATE; PARACETAMOL.

Vertigon (*Smith, Kline & French*) is a proprietary ANTI-EMETIC, available only on prescription, used to relieve symptoms of nausea caused by the vertigo and loss of balance experienced in disorders of the inner and middle ears, or as a result of the administration of CYTOTOXIC drugs in the treatment of cancer. It is produced as spansules (soluble capsules) containing the prochlorperazine (in two strengths).

▲/✚ side-effects/warning: *see* PROCHLORPERAZINE.

Vicks Coldcare (*Richardson-Vicks*) is a proprietary, non-prescription cold relief preparation in the form of capsules, which contain paracetamol, the ANTITUSSIVE dextromethorphan and the decongestant phenylpropanolamine.
▲/✚ side-effects/warning: *see* DEXTROMETHORPHAN; PARACETAMOL.

vigabatrin is an ANTI-EPILEPTIC drug used to treat chronic epilepsy, especially tonic-clonic and partial seizures, when other anti-epileptic drugs are not effective. It is available as tablets.
▲ side-effects: there may be fatigue, dizziness, drowsiness, depression, headache, nervousness and irritability. There are occasional reports of confusion; memory, visual and gastrointestinal disturbances; weight gain; psychoses, and excitation and agitation in children.
✚ warning: administer with caution to patients with kidney impairment, or where there is a history of psychosis or behavioural problems. It should not be given to children under 3 years, or to pregnant or lactating women. Sudden withdrawal should be avoided. Drowsiness may impair skilled performance such as driving.
Related article: SABRIL.

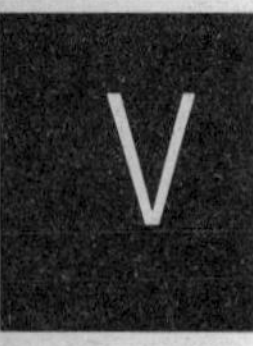

Villescon (*Boehringer Ingelheim*) is a proprietary compound containing the weak STIMULANT prolintane with vitamin supplements; it is used to treat debility or fatigue. Available on prescription only to private patients, it is produced in the form of an elixir.
▲/✚ side-effects/warning: *see* PROLINTANE.

viloxazine is a TRICYCLIC ANTIDEPRESSANT drug that has less of a sedative effect than many. Used to treat depression, dosage must be carefully monitored to remain at an optimum for each individual patient.
▲ side-effects: common effects include sedation (affecting driving ability), dry mouth and blurred vision; there may also be difficulty in urinating, sweating and irregular heartbeat, behavioural disturbances, a rash, a state of confusion, nausea, headache, and/or a loss of libido. Rarely, there are also blood disorders.
✚ warning: viloxazine should not be administered to patients who suffer from heart disease or psychosis; it should be administered with caution to patients who suffer from diabetes, epilepsy, liver or thyroid disease, glaucoma or urinary retention; or who are pregnant or lactating. Withdrawal of treatment must be gradual.
Related article: VIVALAN.

Vivalan (*ICI*) is a proprietary, TRICYCLIC ANTIDEPRESSANT drug, available only on prescription, consisting of tablets containing viloxazine hydrochloride.
▲/✚ side-effects/warning: *see* VILOXAZINE.

Volital (*LAB*) is a proprietary form of the weak STIMULANT pemoline, used to treat hyperactive children. Available only on prescription, it is produced as tablets. It is not recommended for children aged under 6 years.
▲/✚ side-effects/warning: *see* PEMOLINE.

Volraman (*Eastern*) is a proprietary form of the non-steroidal, ANTI-INFLAMMATORY,

non-narcotic, ANALGESIC (NSAID) drug diclofenac sodium. Available on prescription only as tablets (in two strengths) to treat pain and inflammation of musculo-skeletal disorders, such as rheumatic disease.
▲/ ✚ side-effects/warning: *see* DICLOFENAC SODIUM.

Voltarol (*Geigy*) is a proprietary, non-steroid, ANTI-INFLAMMATORY, non-narcotic ANALGESIC, available only on prescription, used to treat arthritic and rheumatic pain and other musculo-skeletal disorders. Its active constituent is diclofenac sodium, and it is produced in the form of tablets (in either of two strengths, plus a sustained-release version called Voltarol Retard), ampoules for injection, and anal suppositories (in either of two strengths). Voltarol should not be administered to patients with a peptic ulcer or asthma, who are known to be allergic to aspirin, or who are pregnant or lactating.
▲/ ✚ side-effects/warning: *see* DICLOFENAC SODIUM.

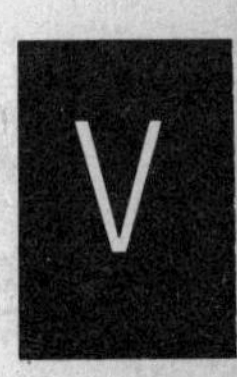

Xanax (*Upjohn*) is a proprietary ANXIOLYTIC, available on prescription only to private patients. It is produced in the form of tablets (in two strengths) containing the BENZODIAZEPINE alprazolam, and is used to treat short-term anxiety and anxiety accompanying depression. Prolonged use may result in dependence.
▲/✚ side-effects/warning: *see* ALPRAZOLAM.

Xylotox (*Astra*) is a proprietary dental local ANAESTHETIC, available only on prescription, containing lignocaine hydrochloride and adrenaline (the latter to add duration to the effect). It is produced in cartridges for easy attachment to a dentist's hypodermic.
▲/✚ side-effects/warning: *see* LIGNOCAINE.

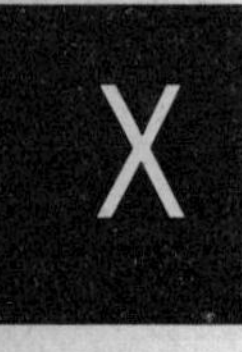

Zarontin (*Parke-Davis*) is a proprietary form of the ANTICONVULSANT drug ethosuximide, available only on prescription, used to treat and suppress petit mal ('absence') seizures. Available in the form of capsules and an elixir for dilution – the potency of the dilute elixir is retained for 14 days – monitoring of seizures following the initiation of treatment with Zarontin should establish an optimum treatment level.

▲/✚ side-effects/warning: *see* ETHOSUXIMIDE.

Zimofane (*Rhône-Poulenc*) is a proprietary form of the HYPNOTIC drug zopiclone. Available on prescription in the form of tablets.

▲/✚ side-effects/warning: *see* ZOPICLONE.

Zofran (*Glaxo*) is a recently introduced ANTI-EMETIC drug, and is a proprietary form of ondansetron, available only on prescription, which gives relief from nausea and vomiting, especially in patients receiving radiotherapy and chemotherapy, and where other drugs are ineffective. It acts by preventing the action of the naturally-occuring hormone and NEUROTRANSMITTER serotonin. It is used in those over 4 years of age, and is available as tablets or in ampoules for administration by slow intravenous injection or infusion

▲/✚ side-effects/warning: *see* ONDANSETRON.

zopiclone is a HYPNOTIC drug for short-term treatment of insomnia. Although it is not a benzodiazepine it causes its hypnotic effect by a similar mechanism. Administration is in the form of tablets. It may cause dependence.

▲ side-effects: there may be drowsiness the next day, which may affect skilled tasks such as driving. The effects of alcohol may be enhanced. There may also be gastrointestinal upsets, irritability, confusion, a depressed mood, light-headedness, rashes, urticaria, hallucinations, loss of memory, and behavioural disturbances. It may also leave a bitter or metallic aftertaste.

✚ warning: zopiclone should not be administered to patients who are pregnant or lactating, or have liver damage, psychiatric illness, or a history of drug abuse.

Related article: ZIMOVANE.

zuclopenthixol is an ANTIPSYCHOTIC drug, one of the thioxanthenes (which resemble in their general actions the phenothiazines such as chlorpromazine), used to treat and restrain psychotic patients, particularly more aggressive or agitated schizophrenic patients. It is available as zuclopenthixol acetate, zuclopenthixol dihydrochloride and zuclopenthixol decanate, in a variety of preparations for administration in the form of tablets, injections, or depot injections.

▲ side-effects: extrapyramidal motor symptoms may occur (muscle spasms, restlessness and tremor), and with prolonged high dosage tardive dyskinesias are possible. There may also be hypothermia, drowsiness, lethargy, insomnia and depression; low blood pressure and heartbeat irregularities; allergic symptoms; and/or dry mouth, constipation, blurred vision, rashes and difficulties in urinating. Prolonged high dosage may cause eventual eye defects and pigmentation of the skin.

✚ warning: zuclopenthixol should not be administered to

Z

patients with heart disease, respiratory disease, epilepsy, parkinsonism, severe arteriosclerosis or acute infection; who are in a withdrawn or apathetic state; who are pregnant or lactating; who have impaired functioning of the liver or kidneys; whose prostate gland is enlarged; who are old and infirm. Withdrawal of treatment must be gradual.

Related article: CLOPIXOL.

Z